RHIT Practice Exam Bundle

2017 Edition

Medical Coding Pro
Copyright © 2017 Medical Coding Pro
All rights reserved.

ISBN-10: 1541039505
ISBN-13: 978-1541039506

DEDICATION

To the hard working students preparing for the RHIT certification exam. Your work ethic and dedication to the medical industry will ensure its health and competency for years to come!

Copyright 2017 Medical Coding Pro
Published by: IPC Marketing LLC
748 Squirrel Hill Dr.
Youngstown, Ohio 44512

ALL RIGHTS RESERVED. No part of this book may be reproduced or transmitted in any form whatsoever, electronic, or mechanical, including photocopying, recording, or by any informational storage or retrieval system without the expressed written, dated and signed permission from the author.

DISCLAIMER AND/OR LEGAL NOTICES:

The information presented herein represents the view of the author as of the date of publication. The book is for informational purposes only.

While every attempt has been made to verify the information provided in this book, neither the author nor his affiliates/partners assume any responsibility for errors, inaccuracies or omissions or for any damages related to use or misuse of the information provided in the book.

Any slights of people or organizations are unintentional. If advice concerning medical or related matters is needed, the services of a fully qualified professional should be sought. Any reference to any person or business whether living or dead is purely coincidental.

Dear Customer,

Thank you for your purchase at Medical Coding Pro! We appreciate the trust you have placed in us to help you with your exam preparation.

As a way of showing our appreciation we have created a DVD called "**Exam Secrets**" and we would like to send it to you **FREE!**

All that we ask is that you email us your feedback that best describes your thoughts on our product. It doesn't matter if the feedback is good or not, we want to hear from you! Your feedback helps a small business like us compete with larger companies by adding a positive review or by telling us how we can improve the product.

Just email us at **freedvd@medicalcodingpro.com** with FREE DVD in the subject line and the following information:

1) The name of the product you purchased.
2) Your product rating on a scale of 1-5, with 5 being the highest.
3) Your feedback. Good feedback might include how our material helped you and what helped you the most.
4) Your full name and shipping address where you would like us to send your FREE DVD.

Thanks again!

Sincerely,

Gregg Zban
Owner/ President
Medical Coding Pro

PROPERTY OF MEDICAL CODING PRO UNAUTHORIZED DISTRIBUTION PROHIBITED SINGLE COPY LICENSE

Quick Start Guide 5

RHIT Overview 6

Basic Housekeeping 8

Keys to Passing the RHIT Exam 9

RHIT Exam Content Outline 15

RHIT Mock Exam Questions 26

RHIT Mock Exam - Answers......................................70

Scoring Sheets 91

Secrets To Reducing Exam Stress............................115

Common Anatomical Terminology 142

Medical Terminology Prefix, Root, and Suffixes........147

Notes 160

Resources 164

Quick Start Guide

Start by reviewing everything included inside the RHIT Practice Exam Bundle. Contents include the following:

1) RHIT Overview
2) Basic Housekeeping
3) Keys To Passing The RHIT Exam
4) RHIT Exam Content Outline
5) RHIT Mock Practice Exam Questions & Answers
6) Scoring Sheets
7) Secrets To Reducing Exam Stress
8) Common Anatomical Terminology
9) Medical Terminology Prefixes, Roots, and Suffixes
10) Notes
11) Resources

These resources will give you a good base to prepare for the certification exam.

If you have any questions please email contact us at
support@medicalcodingpro.com.

Thank you for your business!
Best regards,

Gregg Zban
Medical Coding Pro

RHIT Overview

Registered Health Information Technician (RHIT®)

Professionals holding the RHIT credential are health information technicians who:

- Ensure the quality of medical records by verifying their completeness, accuracy, and proper entry into computer systems.
- Use computer applications to assemble and analyze patient data for the purpose of improving patient care or controlling costs.
- Often specialize in coding diagnoses and procedures in patient records for reimbursement and research. An additional role for RHITs is cancer registrars - compiling and maintaining data on cancer patients.

With experience, the RHIT credential holds solid potential for advancement to management positions, especially when combined with a bachelor's degree.

Although most RHITs work in hospitals, they are also found in other healthcare settings including office-based physician practices, nursing homes, home health agencies, mental health facilities, and public health agencies. In fact, RHITs may be employed in any organization that uses patient data or health information, such as pharmaceutical companies, law and insurance firms, and health product vendors.

Eligibility Requirements

RHIT applicants must meet one of the following eligibility requirements:

- Successfully complete the academic requirements, at an associate's degree level, of an HIM program accredited by the Commission on Accreditation for Health Informatics and Information Management Education (CAHIIM)

OR

- Graduate from an HIM program approved by a foreign association with which AHIMA has a reciprocity agreement[1]

The academic qualifications of each candidate will be verified before a candidate is deemed eligible to take the examination. All first-time applicants must submit an official transcript from their college or university. Early Testing

Students in CAHIIM-accredited programs for RHIT or RHIA®, enrolled in their final term of study, are now eligible to apply for and take their respective certification exam early. Eligible students include the following:

- Students currently enrolled and in their last term of study
- Students who have completed their course work but have not yet graduated
- Graduates that are currently waiting for their official transcripts

source: AHIMA.org

Basic Housekeeping

First lets review some general, but very important, items included in the AHIMA Candidate Guide. You should review the entire guide thoroughly, but here are some important highlights.

Eligibility: Successfully complete an associate level degree in HIM (Health Information Management) OR graduate from an approve HIM program.

Application: Name on the application MUST match the name on your ID's that you will present at the testing center AND your Authorization To Test (ATT) letter. Submit eligibility verification with full payment.

Scheduling: After approval you will receive an (ATT) letter via email. You then have four months from the date on the ATT letter to schedule the exam through Pearson VUE. If you do not take the exam within four months you forfeit your exam fee!

Exam Day: You must arrive at the testing center at least 30 minutes prior to your testing time. If you arrive 15 minutes after your scheduled time you will not be permitted to test and you will forfeit your exam fee! Two forms of ID are required, one with a picture and signature and the other with your signature. These MUST match the name on your ATT letter or you will not be permitted to test.

Exam Scoring: The exam is scored using scaled scoring. Scaled scoring weights the difficulty of each question. Simple questions are given less weigh and more difficult ones are given more weight. Thus each exam, though the questions may be different, will have a passing scaled score of 300 out of 400 based on the difficulty or simplicity of each question.

Now that the basics for the RHIT exam are out of the way, lets take a look how to prepare to pass the exam!

PROPERTY OF MEDICAL CODING PRO UNAUTHORIZED DISTRIBUTION PROHIBITED SINGLE COPY LICENSE

Keys to Passing the RHIT Exam

All students study the information to prepare to take the RHIT exam. It is part of the preparation process for any exam. And while knowing the information is essential, knowing HOW to pass the exam can be just as important.

You do not need 400 out of 400 to pass the exam. You do not have to be "perfect". You just have to be good enough to pass. You only need 300 out of 400 (scaled scoring) to get your certification. That leaves some margin for error and how you manage that margin could be the difference between passing and going back to the drawing board.

Example: You know the answers to 60-70 percent of the questions just from studying the material. The first time through the exam you answer 90 to 100 questions with confidence. How you manage the other 50-60 questions will determine whether you pass the exam or not.

Again, you do not have to be "perfect" on the exam. Just answer enough questions correctly to get your certification.

That is where the following "keys", or tips, on HOW to pass the exam can be extremely valuable to you. I dare say they are just as important to passing the exam as knowing the information.

Knowing one without the other is like taking the exam with one eye closed. You could do it and you might pass, but why chance it when knowing both the information PLUS strategies on how to pass the exam can increase your chances substantially.

How many people have you seen comment on social media or in forums saying they missed getting their certification by a few percentage points? Probably quit a few. I know I see many comments like this. If they only had the information included in the following pages it could have made the difference between passing and failing. Use every advantage, every tip, and it could make the difference for you too.

Key #1: Study and Preparation.

Don't let anyone fool you into thinking that you don't have to study. That is not the case. You NEED to study, and study hard! There are no shortcuts to passing the exam. You must know the material. So put in the time and be prepared! Get as many practice exam questions as you can. The more you get used to answering exam questions the more confident you will be in your ability come exam time. There are 150 questions included in this book. Use them to get used to answering exam question. You can get more practice exam questions at RHITReady.com.

Key #2: Set Up A Study Schedule.

Don't procrastinate! Set up a study schedule that is at least six to eight weeks in advance of taking the exam. Do this now! Set specific days and times to study. Don't just leave it to chance or when you are not busy. You will always find something to do instead of studying. Set times and dates for study and make it part of your routine. You will feel much more relaxed and confident with six to eight weeks of practice under your belt than just leaving it to chance.

Study in two hour increments and no longer. Research shows that after two hours of studying your retention level falls significantly. Schedule two hours per day and stick to it. DO NOT CRAM FOR THE EXAM! You will stress yourself out and won't be able to think clearly during the exam. Study on a daily basis and for a couple hours at the most, then close the books and do something else. If you need a practice schedule planner you can download one here: http://rhitready.com/my-schedule/

Key #3: Study With A Partner or Group.

When possible, study with a partner or in a group. Each of us have strengths and weaknesses. Your strengths may be another persons weaknesses, and their strengths could be your weaknesses. This will help grow your knowledge of the material. Plus, you can share test taking tips as well. this will also serve as a way to make certain you study. It is much more difficult to say no to a study partner or group when you don't feel like studying than saying no to yourself. You can help them put in the time and they will help you.

The knowledge of a group is always larger than the knowledge of a single person. Use that knowledge to help yourself and help others in the process. Strength in numbers!

Key #4: Progress In Segments.

Don't try to do too much right from the start. It can be overwhelming and lower your self confidence, drive, and excitement about getting certified. Take it a step at a time. Start out answering practice questions. Divide the 150 question practice exam included in this guide into three sections.

First 50 Questions: Work through the first 50 questions and take as much time as you need. Don't worry about how long it takes. Just begin by relaxing and answering the practice questions correctly. It doesn't matter if it takes two hours or more to answer them, take your time and get them right. This is the first step and it will help you build your confidence.

Second 50 Questions: Next, after you have spent several practice sessions answering questions without a time limit. Answer the next section of questions with a timer. Give yourself up to two minutes per question. This will be five hours for 150 questions, and certainly not our goal, but it is a good starting point. Keep shortening the time each session until you are below 3 hours and 30 minutes.

Third 50 Questions: Finally, on the last group of questions use the "keys" to help you get through the questions faster. Time yourself too. You should find that your confidence is growing and so is your ability to answer questions correctly and more rapidly.

Key #5: Two Complete Passes through the Exam.

During the exam you want to make TWO passes through the entire exam. The first pass is to answer the easier questions and the second pass is to answer the more difficult ones. Many people do not pass the exam because they get hung up on a few difficult questions in the beginning or middle of the exam and end up running out of time and not answering all the questions. Or worse yet, panicking and rushing through the final 20 or 30 questions while randomly choosing an answer. You will see below there is a method for answering questions that you do not know the answer to. Randomly selecting answers will not give you the BEST chance to get them right. The method below will. Please follow this "key" as it is your path to success.

Key #6: Answer The "First Pass" Questions in One Minute or Less.

Start by making a first pass through the exam. During the first pass through the exam, answer all the questions that you can complete in a reasonable amount of time (one minute or less). If you can't answer the question in one minute, mark it and move on! Practice this technique during your exam preparation so you get used to it.

Key #7: Answer the "Second Pass" Questions in Two Minutes.

After you complete the first pass through the exam, go back and answer the more difficult questions. This time through the exam you can take more time to thoroughly review each exam question and the possible answers. Try to eliminate incorrect answers to increase your chance of selecting the correct answer. Then, carefully direct the remaining answers to see which on best answers the question.

PROPERTY OF MEDICAL CODING PRO UNAUTHORIZED DISTRIBUTION PROHIBITED SINGLE COPY LICENSE

Hopefully you know all the answers, But there is a good chance you will not know all of them. This is where Key #8 comes in…

Key #8: Guessing is a science.

Some guides suggest a guess should be a random choice. I do not agree. Why? Because even though the correct answer might not stare you in the face, chances are you will be able to eliminate at least one, if not more, of the incorrect answers. This will greatly increase your chances to "guess" the correct answer.

Example: There are four multiple choice answers. If you guess randomly you have a 25% chance of guessing correctly. If you can eliminate just one incorrect answer, with certainty, and you guess from the remaining three answers your chances of "guessing" correctly now increase to 33%. Now you have a one in three chance of "guessing" correctly. Eliminate two answers and the percentages go up to a 50% chance of guessing the correct answer. You should never randomly guess unless you have no idea whether ANY of the answers are incorrect or correct. Then close your eyes and pick one.

Key #9: Identify your weaknesses and practice, practice, practice!

Go through each domain and answer questions. Mark down the results and identify your strengths and weaknesses. Spend your study time proportional to your weakest domain to your strongest domain. Know what you know and what you don't and allocate your practice time accordingly.

Bonus Tips:

1. Create a positive, quiet, comfortable study environment.
2. Double check all your work.
3. Do not study more than two hours at a time. You will retain less information after the two hour mark.
4. Select correct answers by eliminating incorrect answers.
5. DO NOT CRAM THE NIGHT BEFORE THE EXAM! This is a recipe for disaster and will cause undue stress.
6. Review the exam registration process.
7. Begin exam preparation at least six to eight weeks prior to the exam.
8. Bring your drivers license and at least one additional form of ID to the testing location and make sure the names on your ID's match what is on the registration.
9. Study in groups. This will keep you engaged and make certain you study even when you don't feel like it.
10. ***KEEP MOVING, KEEP MOVING, AND KEEP MOVING!***

RHIT Exam Content Outline

Number of Questions on Exam:

150 multiple-choice questions (130 scored/ 20 pretest)

Exam Time: 3.5 hours. Any breaks taken will count against your exam time

DOMAIN 1 - Data Analysis and Management (18-22% of overall score)

Tasks:

1. Abstract information found in health records (i.e., coding, research, physician deficiencies, etc.)

2. Analyze data (i.e., productivity reports, quality measures, health record documentation, case mix index

3. Maintain filing and retrieval systems for health records

4. Identify anomalies in data

5. Resolve risks and/or anomalies of data findings

6. Maintain the master patient index (i.e., enterprise systems, merge/ unmerge medical record numbers, etc.)

7. Eliminate duplicate documentation

8. Organize data into a useable format

9. Review trends in data

10. Gather/compile data from multiple sources

11. Generate reports or spreadsheets (i.e., customize, create, etc.)

12. Present data findings (i.e., study results, delinquencies, conclusion/ summaries, gap analysis, graphical

13. Implement workload distribution

14. Design workload distribution

15. Participate in the data management plan (i.e., determine data elements, assemble components, set time-frame)

16. Input and/or submit data to registries

17. Summarize findings from data research/analysis

18. Follow data archive and backup policies

19. Develop data management plan

20. Calculate healthcare statistics (i.e., occupancy rates, length of stay, delinquency rates, etc)

21. Determine validation process for data mapping

22. Maintain data dictionaries

DOMAIN 2 - Coding (16-20% of overall score)

Tasks:

1. Apply all official current coding guidelines

2. Assign diagnostic and procedure codes based on health record documentation

3. Ensure physician documentation supports coding

4. Validate code assignment

5. Abstract data from health record

6. Sequence codes

7. Query physician when additional clinical documentation is needed

8. Review and resolve coding edits (i.e. correct coding initiative, outpatient code editor, NCD, LCD, etc.)

9. Review the accuracy of abstracted data

10. Assign POA (present on admission) indicators

11. Provide educational updates to coders

12. Validate grouper assignment (i.e. MS-DRG, APC, etc.)

13. Identify HAC (hospital acquired condition)

14. Develop and manage a query process

15. Create standards for coding productivity and quality

16. Develop educational guidelines for provider documentation

17. Perform concurrent audits

DOMAIN 3 - Compliance (14-18% of overall score)

Tasks:

1. Ensure patient record documentation meets state and federal regulations

2. Ensure compliance with privacy and security guidelines (HIPAA, state, hospital, etc.)

3. Control access to health information

4. Monitor documentation for completeness

5. Develop a coding compliance plan (i.e., current coding guidelines)

6. Manage release of information

7. Perform continual updates to policies and procedures

8. Implement internal and external audit guidelines

9. Evaluate medical necessity (CDMP – clinical documentation management program)

10. Collaborate with staff to prepare the organization for accreditation, licensing, and/or certification surveys

11. Evaluate medical necessity (Outpatient services)

12. Evaluate medical necessity (Data management)

13. Responding to fraud and abuse

14. Evaluate medical necessity (ISSI (utilization review))

15. Develop forms (i.e., chart review, documentation, EMR, etc.)

16. Evaluate medical necessity (Case management)

17. Analyze access audit trails

18. Ensure valid healthcare provider credentials

DOMAIN 4 - Information Technology (10-14% of overall score)

Tasks:

1. Train users on software

2. Maintain database

3. Set up secure access

4. Evaluate the functionality of applications

5. Create user accounts

6. Trouble-shoot HIM software or support systems

7. Create database

8. Perform end user audits

9. Participate in vendor selection

10. Perform end user needs analysis

11. Design data archive and backup policies

12. Perform system maintenance of software and systems

13. Create data dictionaries

DOMAIN 5 - Quality (10-14% of overall score)

Tasks:

1. Audit health records for content, completeness, accuracy, and timeliness

2. Apply standards, guidelines, and/or regulations to health records

3. Implement corrective actions as determined by audit findings (internal and external)

4. Design efficient workflow processes

5. Comply with national patient safety goals

6. Analyze standards, guidelines, and/or regulations to build criteria for audits

7. Apply process improvement techniques

8. Provide consultation to internal and external users of health information on HIM subject matter

9. Develop reports on audit findings

10. Perform data collection for quality reporting (core measures, PQRI, medical necessity, etc.)

11. Use trended data to participate in performance improvement plans/ initiatives

12. Develop a tool for collecting statistically valid data

13. Conduct clinical pertinence reviews

14. Monitor physician credentials to practice in the facility

RHIT Practice Exam Bundle 2017   23

DOMAIN 6 - Legal (9-13% of overall score)

Tasks:

1. Ensure confidentiality of the health records (paper and electronic)

2. Adhere to disclosure standards and regulations (HIPAA privacy, HITECH Act, breach notifications, etc.) at both state and federal levels

3. Demonstrate and promote legal and ethical standards of practice

4. Maintain integrity of legal health record according to organizational bylaws, rules and regulations

5. Follow state mandated and/or organizational record retention and destruction policies

6. Serve as the custodian of the health records (paper or electronic)

7. Respond to Release of Information (ROI) requests from internal and external requestors

8. Work with risk management department to provide requested documentation

9. Identify potential health record related risk management issues through auditing

10. Respond to and process patient amendment requests to the health record

11. Facilitate basic education regarding the use of consents, healthcare Power of Attorney, Advanced Directives, DNRs, etc.

12. Represent the facility in court related matters as it applies to the health record (subpoenas, depositions, court orders, warrants)

PROPERTY OF MEDICAL CODING PRO UNAUTHORIZED DISTRIBUTION PROHIBITED SINGLE COPY LICENSE

DOMAIN 7 - Revenue Cycle (9-13% of overall score)

Tasks:

1. Communicate with providers to discuss documentation deficiencies (i.e. queries)

2. Participate in clinical documentation improvement programs to ensure proper documentation of health records

3. Collaborate with other departments on monitoring accounts receivable (i.e. unbilled, uncoded)

4. Provide ongoing education to healthcare providers (i.e. regulatory changes, new guidelines, payment standards, best practices, etc)

5. Identify fraud and abuse

6. Assist with appeal letters in response to claim denials

7. Monitor claim denials/over-payments to identify potential revenue impact

8. Prioritize the work according to accounts receivable, patient type, etc.

9. Distribute the work according to accounts receivable, patient type, etc.

10. Maintain the chargemaster

11. Ensure physicians are credentialed with different payers for reimbursement

Source: AHIMA.org website

RHIT Mock Practice Exam - Questions & Answers
2017 Edition

The following is an RHIT Mock Practice Exam. You may not use any outside materials for this exam other than the manuals referenced by the American Health Information Management Association (AHIMA).

To pass the certification exam you must manage your time carefully. Time is the single most controllable factor by students and time mismanagement is one of the major reasons student fail the exam.

A Registered Health Information Technician is an individual of high professional integrity who has passed an RHIT certification examination.

Exam Details:

Questions:
150 multiple-choice questions (130 scored/ 20 pretest).

Time:
3 hours and 30 minutes. Any breaks taken will be counted against your exam time.

Fee:
$299 non AHIMA members
$229 AHIMA members

RHIT Mock Exam Questions

Domain 1 - Data Analysis and Management (30 Questions)

1. In designing a new form or computer view, the designer should be most driven by?

a. Needs of the users
b. What information should be coded
c. Authors of entries in a health record
d. Needs of the patients

2. What data entry software system do home health agencies use?

a. incidence-only population-based registry
b. Home Health Agency
c. HAVEN (Home Assessment Validation and Entry)
d. A release of information company

3. Which rate is used to compare the number of inpatient deaths to the total number of inpatient deaths and discharges?

a. Net hospital death rate
b. Fetal/newborn/maternal hospital death rate
c. Gross hospital death rate
d. Adjusted hospital death rate

4. In a problem oriented health record, problems are organized...

a. In alphabetical order
b. In numeric order
c. By date of onset
d. Non of the above

5. A health information technician is responsible for designing a data collection form to collect data on patients in an acute care hospital. The first resource that should be used is:

a. UHDDS
b. UACDS
c. MDS
d. ORYS

6. In long term care the residents care plan is based on data collected in what system?

a. UHDDS
b. OASIS
c. MDS
d. HEIDS

7. Which of the following is NOT a characteristic of high quality healthcare?

a. Data relevancy
b. Data currency
c. Data consistency
d. Data accountability

8. The RHIT supervisor for the filing and retrial section of Community Clinic is developing a staffing schedule for the year. The clinic is open 260 days per year and has an average of 500 clinic visits per day. The standard for filing records is 50 per hour. For retrieving records it is 40 per hour. How many filing hours will be required daily to retrieve and file records for each clinic day?

a. 10 Hours per day
b. 11.11 Hours per day
c. 12.5 Hours per day
d. 22.5 Hours per day

PROPERTY OF MEDICAL CODING PRO UNAUTHORIZED DISTRIBUTION PROHIBITED SINGLE COPY LICENSE

9. Term used to articulate the number of inpatients present at any one time in a healthcare facility?

a. Average daily census
b. Census
c. Inpatient service day
d. Length of stay

10. Which of the following materials is NOT documented in an emergency record?

a. Time and means of patient arrival
b. Patients instruction at discharge
c. Patients complete medical history
d. Emergency care administered before arrival at the facility

11. What is the difference between data and information?

a. Data represents basic facts, information provides meaning
b. Data is expressed in numbers, information is expressed in words
c. Information must be kept confidential, data can be shared
d. Information is about people, data is about things

12. Which term is used to describe the number of inpatients present at the census taking time each day PLUS the number of patients that were both admitted and discharged after the census taking time the previous day?

a. Inpatient occupancy rate
b. Bed count
c. Average Daily Census
d. Daily inpatient census

13. Which rate describes the probability of occurrence of a medical condition in a population over a period of time?

a. Mortality
b. Morbidity
c. Incidence
d. Prevalence

14. Patient care managers use the data and information documented in the health record to

a. Evaluate patterns and trends in patient care
b. Provide direct patient care
c. Generate patient bills and third party claims for reimbursement
d. Determine the extent and effect of occupational hazards.

15. An outpatient clinic is reviewing the functionality of an EHR it is considering purchasing. Which of the following data sets should the clinic consult to ensure that all of the federally recommended data elements for Medicare and Medicaid outpatients are collected by the system?

a. DEEDA
b. EMEDS
c. UACDS
d. UHDDS

16. The HIM department recently performed an audit of health records. The audit showed that for the 10,000 records filed there was a 7 percent error rate. The national average of each misfile is $200. What is the labor cost for the department for handling these misfiled reports?

a. $1,400
b. $14,000
c. $140,000
d. $285,714

17. The Home Health Prospective Payment System (HHPPS) uses the _____ data set for patient assessments.

a. UHDDS
b. OASIS
c. HCPCS
d. MDS

18. The Outcome and Assessment Information Set (OASIS) data are used to assess the _____ of home health services.

a. Quality
b. Accuracy
c. Outcome
d. Objective

19. The data set designed to organize data for public release about the outcomes of care is _____?

a. HEDIS
b. UHDDS
c. MDS
d. HCPCS

20. In Long Term Care "LTC", the resident's care plan is based on data collected in the _____?

a. MDS Version 2.0
b. Data Dictionary
c. NCHS
d. None of the above

21. Which of the following provides a standardized vocabulary for facilitating the development of computer-based records?

a. HCPCS
b. UHDDS
c. OASIS
d. HEDIS

22. Community Hospital has 250 patients in the hospital at midnight on May 1st. They admit 30 patients on May 2nd. The hospital discharged 40 patients, including deaths, on May 2nd. Two patients were both admitted and discharged on May 2nd. What is the total number of inpatient service days for May 2nd?

a. 240
b. 242
c. 280
d. 320

23. Community Hospital has more than 100 clinical databases. The Data Quality Committee is studying the comparability among the databases.The data elements and data definitions are cataloged for each database. What would be the next logical step in determining the degree of comparability among the database?

a. Identify the operating system for each database and determine if they are similar to each other.

b. Select a representative set of data elements and track these across the database to identify consistencies and differences.

c. Identify the network capability of each of the databases so that data can be exchanged.

d. Determine the volume and type of data stored within each database so that a repository of similar data can be developed

24. Once hospital discharge abstract systems were developed and their ability to provide comparative data to hospitals was established it became necessary to develop....

a. Data sets
b. Data elements
c. Electronic data interchanged.
d. Bills of mortality

25. Which of the following provides a system for classifying morbidity and mortality information for statistical purposes?

a. CPT
b. DSMMD 4th Edition
c. HCPCS
d. ICD10-CM

26. After the type of cases to be included in a registry have been determined, what is the next step in data acquisition?

a. Registering
b. Defining
c. Abstracting
d. Finding

27. Which of the following use data from the MDS for long term care?

a. Centers for Medicare and Medicaid Services
b. Home health hospice agencies
c. Home health agencies
d. Rehabilitation facilities

28. A Health Record Technician has been asked to review the discharge patient abstracting module of a proposed new EHR. Which of the following data sets would the technician consult to ensure the system collects all federally required discharge data elements for Medicare and Medicaid inpatients in an acute-care hospital?

a. Select a representative set of data elements and track these across the database to identify consistencies and differences.

b. Identify the network repeatability of each of the databases so that the data can be exchanged.

c. Determine the volume and type of data stored within each database so that the repository of similar data can be developed.

d. All of the above.

29. A critical early step in designing an EMR "electronic medical record " is to develop _____ in which the characteristics of each data element are defined.

a. Data currency
b. Data Dictionary
c. Minimum Data Set
d. Classification of patients

30. A core data set developed by the American Society for Testing and Materials (ASTM) to communicate a patient's past and current health information as the patient transitions from one care setting to another is _____?

a. Concept Table
b. Common Data Elements
c. Core Data Elements
d. Continuity of Care Record

Domain 2 - Coding (25 Questions)

31. Coding productivity consists of:

a. Accuracy and volume
b. Accuracy
c. Volume
d. CMI

32. Which of the following codes would be used when coding a hydrocystoma of the right eyelid?

a. D22.11
b. D22.10
c. D23.11
d. D23.12

33. Uniform reporting and statistical data collection for medical procedures, supplies, products, and services are promoted by which of the following?

a. CPT
b. HCPCS
c. ICD-10-CM
d. ICD-10-PCS

34. Which of the following healthcare programs cover dependents and survivors of permanently and totally disabled veterans?

a. CHAMPUS
b. CHAMPVA
c. HIS
d. TRICARE

35. A patient was diagnosed with L4-L5 lumbar neuropathy and discogenic pain. The patient underwent an intradiscal electrothermal annuloplasty (IDET) in the radiology suite. What ICD-10-CM procedure code is used?

a. M47.16
b. M51.26
c. 0S523ZZ
d. 03LY0CZ

36. Which of the following is the most comprehensive controlled vocabulary for coding the content of a patient record?

a. CPT
b. HCPCS
c. ICD-10-CM
d. SNOMED-CT

37. A patient is admitted to the hospital with shortness of breath and congestive heart failure. The patient subsequently develops respiratory failure and is intubated and placed on ventilator management. Which of the following would be the correct code sequencing?

a. Respiratory failure, intubation, ventilator management

b. Congestive heart failure, respiratory failure, ventilator management, intubation

c. Respiratory failure, congestive heart failure, intubation, ventilator management

d. Shortness of breath, congestive heart failure, respiratory failure, ventilator management

38. A patient had a placenta previa with delivery of twins. The patient had two prior Cesarean sections and this C-section was due to hemorrhage. The principal diagnosis would be:

a. Normal delivery
b. Placenta previa
c. Twin gestation
d. Vaginal hemorrhage

39. The APC payment system is based on what coding system?

a. CPT and HCPCS codes
b. ICD-10-CM diagnosis and procedure codes
c. CPT and ICD-10-CM procedure codes
d. Only CPT codes

40. What is the purpose of the present on admission (POA) indicator?

a. Differentiate between conditions present on admission and conditions that develop during an inpatient admission.

b. Track principal diagnoses

c. Distinguish between principal and primary diagnoses.

d.Determine principal diagnosis

41. Which of the following prospective payment systems is utilized for payment of inpatient services?

a. APC
b. DRG
c. OPPS
d. RBRVS

42. A 75 year old male is admitted with fever, lethargy, hypotension, tachycardia, oliguria, and elevated WBC. The patient has more than 100,000 organisms of Escherichia coli per cc of urine. The attending physician documents "urosepsis." How should the coder proceed?

a. Code sepsis as the principal diagnosis and urinary tract infection due to E coli as a secondary diagnosis.

b. Code urinary tract infection with sepsis as the principal diagnosis.

c. Query the physician to ask if the patient has septicemia because of the symptomatology.

d. Query the physician to ask if the patient had septic shock so that this may be used as the principal diagnosis.

43. How is the Medicare benefit period defined?

a. Beginning the day the Medicare patient is admitted to the hospital and ending when the patient has not been hospitalized for a period of sixty consecutive days.

b. The period in which a Medicare patient is hospitalized.

c. The period that begins on January 1 of each year with an allowable inpatient hospitalization benefit up to 90 days.

d. Between one and 90 days of a Medicare patient's hospitalizations.

44. Healthcare cost and lost income associated with work-related injuries is covered by which of the following healthcare?

a. CHAMPVA
b. Medicare
c. Medicaid
d. Workers' compensation

45. The Medicare inpatient prospective payment system excludes which of the following types of hospitals?

a. Children's
b. Rural
c. State supported
d. Tertiary

46. In processing a Medicare payment for outpatient radiology exams a hospital outpatient services department would receive payment under which of the following payment systems?

a. DRGs
b. HHRGS
c. OASIS
d. OPPS

47. Which of the following program provides additional federal funds to states so that Medicaid eligibility can be expanded to include a greater number of children?

a. Medigap
b. PACE
c. SCHIP
d. TRICARE

48. A 50 yo female is admitted with abdominal pain. The physician states that the discharge diagnosis is pancreatitis versus noncalculus cholecystitis. Both diagnoses are treated equally. The correct coding and sequencing of the case would be:

a. Sequence either the pancreatitis or the noncalculus cholecystitis as the principal diagnosis.

b. Pancreatitis; noncalculus cholecystitis; abdominal pain.

c. Noncalculus cholecystitis; pancreatitis; abdominal pain.

d. Abdominal pain; pancreatitis; noncalculus cholecystitis.

49. A patient presents to the doctor's office with fever, productive cough and shortness of breath. The physician orders a chest x-ray and indicates in the progress note: "Rule Out pneumonia"
If the results have not yet been received, what should the coder report for the visit?

a. Pneumonia
b. Fever, cough, shortness of breath
c. Cough, shortness of breath
d. Pneumonia, cough, shortness of breath, fever

50. The following system provides a detailed classification system for coding of the histology, topography, and behavior of neoplasm?

a. Current Procedural Terminology
b. Healthcare Common Procedure Coding System
c. International Classification of Disease for Oncology, Third Edition
d. Systematized Nomenclature of Medicine Clinical Terminology

51. Substance abuse and mental health disorders are collected by which set of codes?

a. CPT
b. DSM-V-TR
c. HCPCS
d. SNOMED CT

52. If a medication list contains the drug Procardia, which of the following diagnosis should the coder find?

a. Hypertension
b. Esophagitis
c. Congestive Heart Failure
d. AIDS

53. Updating the procedure classification of ICD-10-CM is done by which of the following?

a. Centers for Disease Control (CDC)
b. Centers for Medicare and Medicaid Services (CMS)
c. National Center for Health Statistics (NCHS)
d. Combination of all three.

54. In processing a bill under the Medicare outpatient prospective payment system (OPPS), where a patient had three surgical procedures performed during the same operative session, which of the following would apply?

a. Bundling of services
b. Outlier adjustment
c. Pass-through payment
d. Discounting of procedures

55.A patient has carcinoma of multiple overlapping sites of the bladder. A diagnostic cystoscopy and transurethral fulgeration of the bladder lesion (1.9cm, 6.0cm) are undertaken. Which of the following CPT code(s) would be most appropriate?

a. 52234, 52240
b. 52235
c. 52240
d. 52200, 52234, 52240

Domain 3 - Compliance (25 Questions)

56. In preparation for an EHR, you are conducting a total facility inventory of all forms currently used. You must name each form for bar coding and indexing into a document management system. The unnamed document in front of you includes a microscopic description of tissue excised during surgery. The document type you are most likely to give to this form is:

a. Pathology report.
b. Operative report.
c. Discharge summary.
d. Recovery room record.

57. In the past, Joint Commission standards have focused on promoting the use of a facility approved abbreviation list to be used by hospital care providers. With the advent of the Commission's national patient safety goals, the focus has shifted to...

a. use of prohibited or "dangerous" abbreviations.
b. prohibited use of any abbreviations.
c. use of abbreviations used in the final diagnoses.
d. flagrant use of specialty-specific abbreviations.

58. As a trauma registrar working in an emergency department, you want to begin comparing your trauma care services to other hospital-based emergency departments. To ensure that your facility is collecting the same data as other facilities, you review elements from which data set?

a. MDS
b. DEEDS
c. UHDDS
d. ORYX

RHIT Practice Exam Bundle 2017   43

59. Skilled nursing facilities may choose to submit MDS data using RAVEN software, or software purchased commercially through a vendor, provided that the software meets

a. Joint Commission standards.
b. HL-7 standards.
c. CMS standards.
d. NHIN standards.

60. When operating under the Health Insurance Portability and Accountability Act of 1996 (HIPAA), what is a basic tenet in information security for health care professionals to follow?

a. The information system encourages mass copying, printing, and downloading of patient records.

b. Security training is provided to all levels of staff.

c. Patients are not educated about their right to confidentiality of health information.

d. When paper-based records are no longer needed, they are bundled and sent to a recycling center.

61. Medicare's Conditions of Participation for Hospitals requires that patient health records be retained for at least _____ years unless a longer period is required by state or local laws.

a. Seven
b. Five
c. Three
d. Ten

PROPERTY OF MEDICAL CODING PRO UNAUTHORIZED DISTRIBUTION PROHIBITED SINGLE COPY LICENSE

62. Which of the following responsibilities would you expect to find on the job description of a facility's Information Security Officer but NOT on the job description of Chief Privacy Officer?

a. Monitor the facility's business associate agreements.

b. Conduct audit trails to monitor inappropriate access to system information.

c. Cooperate with the Office of Civil Rights in compliance investigations.

d. Oversee the patient's right to inspect, amend, and restrict access to protected health information.

63. What is the best resource to reference for recent certification standards to determine your acute care facility's degree of compliance with prospective payment requirements for Medicare?

a. CARF manual.
b. Joint Commission accreditation manual.
c. Federal Register.
d. Hospital bylaws.

64. Which index is used by the HIM department to link the patients name and number in relation to access and retention of the clinical record?

a. Master patient index
b. Physician index
c. Disease index
d. Operation index

65. Part of the responsibilities of the Health Information Manager (HIM) is to _____

a. Secure the data records for the hospital.

b. Perform background checks on new employees.

c. Educate physicians regarding proper documentation policies and standards.

d. Make sure each employee has the proper certification for their department.

66. In a manual record tracking system, no record should be removed from the file without being replaced by a(n)

a. Outguide
b. 8 1/2 × 11 inch charge-out slip
c. Paddle
d. Empty file folder

67. AHIMA recommends that patient health information for minors be retained for at least how long?

a. Ten years after the age of majority
b. Ten years after the most recent encounter
c. Age of majority plus statute of limitation
d. Permanently

68. The steps in developing a record retention program include all but which one of the following?

a. Destroying records that are no longer needed
b. Notifying the courts of the destruction
c. Assigning each record a retention period
d. Determining the format and location of storage

69. In preparation for an upcoming site visit by Joint Commission, you discover that the number of delinquent records for the preceding month exceeded 50% of discharged patients. Even more alarming was the pattern you noticed in the type of delinquencies. Which of the following represents the most serious pattern of delinquencies? Fifteen percent of delinquent records show

a. Absence of SOAP format in progress notes.
b. Missing signatures on progress notes.
c. Missing operative reports.
d. Missing discharge summaries.

70. According to AHIMA's recommended retention standards, which one of the following types of health information does NOT need to be retained permanently?

a. Register of deaths
b. Register of surgical procedures
c. Register of births
d. Physician index

71. Accreditation by Joint Commission is a voluntary activity for a facility and it is….

a. Required for reimbursement of certain patient groups.
b. Required for state licensure in all states.
c. Considered unnecessary by most health care facilities.
d. Conducted in each facility annually.

72. Your hospital has purchased a number of outpatient facilities. You have been assigned to chair an interdisciplinary committee that will write record retention policies for the new corporation. You begin by telling the committee their primary consideration when making retention decisions must be_____.

PROPERTY OF MEDICAL CODING PRO UNAUTHORIZED DISTRIBUTION PROHIBITED SINGLE COPY LICENSE

a. Provider preferences.
b. Professional standards.
c. Statutory requirements.
d. Space considerations.

73. Engaging patients and their families in health care decisions is one of the core objectives for

a. The Joint Commission's National Patient Safety goals
b. Achieving meaningful use of EHRs
c. HIPAA 5010 regulations
d. Establishing flexible clinical pathways

74. What follow-up rate does the American College of Surgeons mandate for all cancer cases to meet approval requirements as a cancer program?

a. 80%
b. 90%
c. 100%
d. 70%

75. In which registry would you expect to find an Injury Severity Score (ISS)?

a. Birth Defects Registry
b. Cancer Registry
c. Transplant Registry
d. Trauma Registry

76. In 1987, OBRA helped shift the focus in long-term care to patient outcomes. As a result, core assessment data elements are collected on each Skilled Nursing Facility resident as defined in the _____.

a. Uniform Ambulatory Core Data.
b. MDS.
c. UHDDS.
d. Uniform Clinical Data Set.

77. Which method of identification of authorship or authentication of entries would be inappropriate to use in a patient's health record?

a. Delegated use of computer key by radiology secretary.
b. Identifiable initials of a nurse writing a nursing note.
c. A unique identification code entered by the person making the report.
d. Written signature of the provider of care.

78. The health care providers at your hospital do a very thorough job of periodic open record review to ensure the completeness of record documentation. A qualitative review of surgical records would likely include checking for documentation regarding _____.

a. The quality of follow-up care.

b. The presence or absence of such items as preoperative and postoperative diagnosis, description of findings, and specimens removed.

c. Whether the severity of illness and/or intensity of service warranted acute level care.

d. Whether a postoperative infection occurred and how it was treated.

79. Your state regulations require records to be kept for a statute of limitations period of seven years. Federal law requires records to be retained for five years. The minimum retention period for health records in your facility should be

a. Five years
b. Seven years
c. Either five or seven years as determined by the facility
d. Ten years

80. Stage I of meaningful use focuses on data capture and sharing. Which of the following is included in the menu set of objectives for eligible hospitals in this stage?

a. Establish critical pathways for complex, high-dollar cases
b. Appropriate use of HL-7 standards
c. Use CPOE for medication orders
d. Smoking cessation counseling for MI patients

Domain 4 - Information Technologies (20 Questions)

81. Which of the following stores data in predefined tables consisting of rows and columns?

a. Spreadsheet
b. Relational database
c. Hierarchical database
d. Network database

82. Which of the following best describes the function of kiosks?

a. Computer station that physicians can use to order medications.

b. Computer station that facilitates integrated communications within the healthcare organizations.

c. Computer station that unlocks workstations.

d. Computer station that promotes the healthcare organization's services.

83. To ensure that a CPOE system supports patient safety, what other system must also be in practice?

a. Digital dictation
b. Electronic nursing notes
c. Pharmacy information system
d. Point of care charting

84. When some computers are used primarily to enter data and others to process data, this architecture is called?

a. Client/ server
b. LAN
c. Mainframe
d. Web services

85. These standards cover the use of personal ID numbers that restrict the use to a system.

a. Identification
b. Authentication
c. Certification
d. All of the above

86. A transition technology used by many hospitals to increase access to health record content, and receive it as quickly as possible is:

a. EHR
b. EDMS
c. Electronic signature authentication
d. EDI (electronic data interchange)

87. This type of information system would be used for processing patient admissions, employee time cards, and purchase orders; the day-to-day operations of a business.

a. Transaction processing system
b. MIS
c. Decision-processing system
d. Expert System

88. Which of the following would be used to control user access in an EHR?

a. Data definition
b. Relational database
c. Database management system
d. Data mining

89. In which phase of the system's development life cycle is the primary focus on identifying and assigning priorities to the various upgrades and changes that might be made in an organization's information systems?

a. Design
b. Implementation
c. Maintenance
d. Planning

90. Which of the following tasks is not performed in an EHR system?

a. Document imaging
b. Analysis
c. Assembly
d. Indexing

91. Systems testing of a new IS should be conducted using:

a. Data supplied by the vendor
b. Test data
c. Actual patient data
d. Data from the training database

92. The concept of systems integration refers to the healthcare organization's ability to:

a. Combine information from any system within the organization.
b. Use information from one system at a time.
c. Combine information from systems outside the organization.
d. Use information strictly for administrative purposes.

RHIT Practice Exam Bundle 2017
53

93. What is the key piece of data needed to link a patient who is seen in a variety of care settings?

a. Facility medical record number
b. Facility identification number
c. Identity matching algorithm
d. Patient birth data

94. Which of the following is a snapshot in time and consolidates data from multiple sources to enhance decision making?

a. CDW
b. DSS
c. KMS
d. MIS

95. Before purchasing an EHR system, a clinical office practice should consult which of the following to ensure the system meets the HL7 standards for EHR system functionality?

a. CCHIT
b. HIE
c. CMS
d. NCVHS

96. I am looking for a method of data security. Which of the following would be one of my choices?

a. Cryptography
b. Firewall
c. User access
d. All of the above

PROPERTY OF MEDICAL CODING PRO UNAUTHORIZED DISTRIBUTION PROHIBITED SINGLE COPY LICENSE

97. Which of the following security controls are built into a computer software program?

a. Physical safeguards
b. Administration safeguards
c. Application safeguards
d. Media safeguards

98. Which statement is true concerning CDR and EHR.

a. CDR supports management of data for an EHR
b. CDR and an EHR are the same
c. CDR is an early stage of EHR
d. CDR captures documents, EHR captures data

99. Which of the following is a family of standards that aids in the exchange of data among hospital systems and physician practices?

a. CTI
b. LAN
c. HL7
d. WAN

100. One of the advantages of an EDMS is that it can:

a. Help manage work tasks
b. Decrease the time records should be retained
c. Improve communications with physicians
d. Eliminate all of the problems encountered with the paper record

Domain 5 - Quality (20 Questions)

101. During The Utilization Review Committee meeting, a case presented for discussion involved a surgical case resulting in unexpected loss of lower extremity below the knee due to complications requiring extended length of stay. Being a Sentinel event, the committee requested that an investigation and reporting was required to identify the cause and prevention of future occurrences. This investigation and required reporting to the joint commission is known as:

a. Root cause analysis
b. Potential compensable event
c. Medication review
d. Clinical report card

102. After a review of the patients record it was discovered there was no history and physical on the record at seven hours passed this patient's admission time. This would be in a sample of:

a. Quantitative analysis
b. Qualitative analysis
c. Data mining
d. Data warehousing

103. The director wants to implement benchmarking for transcription at a clinic. There are 21 transcriptionists who average about 140 lines per hour. They support 80 physicians at a cost of 15 cents per line. What is the first step the director takes to establish benchmarks for this group?

a. Define what is to be studied and accomplished by instituting benchmarks.

b. Hold a meeting to announce benchmark program.

c. Obtain benchmarks from other institutions.

d. Hire a consultant.

104. In qualitative analysis we ensure documentation supports the diagnosis. What documentation would a coder look for to substantiate the diagnosis of aspiration pneumonia?

a. Diffuse parenchymal lung disease on x-ray
b. Patient history of inhaled food, liquid or oil
c. Positive culture for Pneumocystis carinii
d. Positive culture for Streptococcus pneumonia

105. The United States federal government's Medicare substitutes compliance with the Conditions of Participation requirement to hospitals that already have accreditations awarded by various other agencies that include the Joint Commission, CARF, AOA, or AAAHC. This is known as:

a. Deemed status
b. Due process
c. Contingency statutory
d. Waived status

106. The primary objective of quality in healthcare for both patient and provider is to:

a. Keep costs under control
b. Reduce death rates
c. Reduce the incidence of infectious diseases
d. Arrive at the desired outcomes

107. Which of the following is not a responsibility of an organization's quality management department?

a. Help departments to identify potential clinical quality problems
b. Participating in regular department meetings across the organization
c. Conduct medical peer review to identify patterns of care
d. Determining the method for studying potential problems

108. A coding supervisor who makes up the weekly work schedule would engage in what type of planning?

a. Long-range
b. Operational
c. Tactical
d. Strategic

109. This data set was developed by the National Committee for Quality Assurance to aid consumers with health related issues with information to compare performance of clinical measures for health plans:

a. HEDIS
b. UHDDS
c. UACDS
d. ORYX

110. A key feature of performance improvement is:

a. Replacing unstructured decision making
b. Developing managers to control processes
c. An endless loop of feedback
d. A continuous cycle of improvement

111. The Joint Commission on site survey process incorporates tracer methodology, which emphasizes surveyor review by means of:

a. Patient tracer
b. System tracers
c. Both system and patient tracers
d. Policy and procedure manual reviews

112. In this case management step, the case manager confirms that the patient meets criteria for the care setting and depth of services can be provided at the facility.

a. Pre-admission care planning
b. Care planning at the time of admission
c. Review the progress of care
d. Discharge planning

113. Every organization's risk management plan should include the following components except:

a. Loss prevention and reduction
b. Safety and security management
c. Peer review
d. Claims management

114. A standard of performance or best practice for a particular process or outcome is called a(n):

a. Performance measure
b. Benchmark
c. Improvement opportunity
d. Data measure

115. A patient satisfaction survey conducted post discharge is a method of quality measure through:

a. Prospective indicator
b. Structured indicator
c. Process indicator
d. Outcome indicator

116. Which of the following is not a step in quality improvement decision-making?

a. Determination of the quickest solution
b. Definition of the problem
c. Development of alternative solutions
d. Implementation and follow-up

117. The goal of non-financial chart audits?

a. Find the root cause of a problem
b. Prepare for a quarterly meeting
c. Quality improvement
d. Avoid an OIG audit

118. Who is responsible for ensuring the quality of health record documentation?

a. Board of directors
b. Administrator
c. Providers
d. HIM professionals

119. Change management is the process of planning for change. It concentrates on:

a. Addressing employee resistance to change
b. Scheduling planned changes
c. Implementing the technology to execute changes
d. Managing the costs of changes

120. Where is Six Sigma used?

a. Where very large deviations can have an insignificant impact.
b. Where very small deviations can have a significant impact.
c. Where all other cost saving measure have failed.
d. After Five Sigma.

Domain 6 - Legal (15 Questions)

121. Which of the following statements is true about a requested restriction?

a. ARRA states that a CE does not have to agree to a requested restriction.

b. ARRA mandates that a CE must comply with a requested restriction unless it meets one of the exceptions.

c. ARRA mandates that a CE must comply with a requested restriction.

d. ARRA does not address restrictions to PHI.

122. You have been assigned the responsibility of performing an audit to confirm that all of the workforce's access is appropriate for their role in the organization. This process is called_____?

a. Information access management.
b. Risk assessment.
c. Information system activity review.
d. Workforce clearance procedure.

123. A patient has submitted an authorization to release information to a physician office for continued care. The release of information clerk wants to limit the information provided because of the minimum necessary rule. What should the supervisor tell the clerk?

a. The minimum necessary rule was eliminated with ARRA.
b. Good call.
c. The patient is an exception to the minimum necessary rule so process the request as written.
d. The minimum necessary rule only applies to attorneys.

PROPERTY OF MEDICAL CODING PRO UNAUTHORIZED DISTRIBUTION PROHIBITED SINGLE COPY LICENSE

124. An HIM educator speaks on department design and the legislative act or agency that was created to ensure that workers have a safe and healthy work environment. Which of the following topics will be discussed?

a. OSH Act
b. Wagner Act
c. Labor Management Relations Act
d. Taft-Hartley Law

125. A patient asked to view her medical record. The record is stored off-site. How long does the facility have to provide this record to him?

a. 60 days
b. 30 days
c. 14 days
d. 10 days

126. One of the responsibilities of a Chief Privacy Officer for a hospital is to _____.

a. Develop a plan for reporting privacy complaints
b. Back up data
c. Writing policies on protecting hardware
d. Writing policies on encryption standards

127. Employers may be able to demonstrate that age is a reasonable requirement for a position. Such an exception to the Age Discrimination Employment Act (ADEA) is called _____?

a. Bona fide occupational qualification.
b. Job description essential.
c. Essential element for employment.
d. There is no such exception to ADEA.

128. Laws that limits the time period during which legal action may be brought against another party are known as _____?

a. Case law
b. Summons
c. Common law
d. Statutes of limitations

129. Which of the following HIPAA components would the general New Employee Orientation training most likely cover?

a. Physical/ workstation security
b. Job-specific training (e.g., patient's right to amend record)
c. Business associate agreements
d. Marketing issues

130. A surgeon comes out to speak to a patient's family. He tells them the patient came through the surgery fine. The mass was benign and they could see the patient in an hour. He talks low so that the other people in the waiting room will not hear but someone walked by and heard. This is called a(n)

a. Violation of policy
b. Privacy breach
c. Incidental disclosure
d. Privacy incident

131. A manager just identified that an employee looked up his own medical record. Which of the following actions should be taken?

a. Follow the incident response procedure.
b. Terminate the employee on the spot.
c. Notify OCR.
d. Notify his or her supervisor because this is a minor incident and therefore not subject to the incident response procedure.

132. What is the difference between an Institutional Review Board (IRB) and a hospital's Ethics Committee?

a. The IRB deals with the ethical treatment of human research subjects, and the Ethics Committee covers a wide range of issues.

b. The IRB focuses on patient care only, and the Ethics Committee addresses both patient care and business practices.

c. The Ethics Committee reviews ethics complaints, and the IRB focuses on developing policies and procedures.

d. The IRB is made up entirely of patient care providers, and the Ethics Committee is multidisciplinary.

133. When developing a record retention policy, the HIM professionals should consider all of the following EXCEPT _____.

a. All applicable statutes and regulations
b. The thickness of the records
c. Uses of and need for information
d. Current storage space

134. In general, which of the following statements is correct?

a. When federal and state laws conflict, valid corporate policies supersede federal and state laws.

b. When federal and state laws conflict, valid federal laws supersede state laws.

c. When federal and state laws conflict, valid state laws supersede federal laws.

d. When federal and state laws conflict, valid local laws supersede federal and state laws.

135. Which of the following would be an inappropriate procedure for the custodian of the medical record to perform prior to taking a medical record from a health care facility to court?

a. Document in the file folder the total number of pages in the record.
b. Prepare an itemized list of sheets contained in the medical record.
c. Number each page of the record in ink.
d. Remove any information that might prove detrimental to the hospital or physician.

Domain 7 - Revenue Cycle (15 Questions)

136. All of the following items are "packaged" under the Medicare outpatient prospective payment system, EXCEPT for _____.

a. Medical visits
b. Medical supplies
c. Recovery room
d. Anesthesia

137. A patient with Medicare is seen in the physician's office. The total charge for this office visit is $250.00. The patient has previously paid his deductible under Medicare Part B. The PAR Medicare fee schedule amount for this service is $200.00. The nonPAR Medicare fee schedule amount for this service is $190.00. If this physician is a participating physician who accepts assignment for this claim, the total amount the physician will receive is

a. $250.00.
b. $190.00.
c. $218.50.
d. $200.00.

138. A computer software program that assigns appropriate MS-DRGs according to the information provided for each episode of care is called a(n)_____.

a. Scrubber.
b. Case-mix analyzer.
c. Encoder.
d. Grouper.

PROPERTY OF MEDICAL CODING PRO UNAUTHORIZED DISTRIBUTION PROHIBITED SINGLE COPY LICENSE

139. This accounting method attributes a dollar figure to every input required to provide a service.

a. Reimbursement
b. Cost accounting
c. Charge accounting
d. Contractual allowance

140. The term used to indicate that the service or procedure is reasonable and necessary for the diagnosis or treatment of illness or injury consistent with generally accepted standards of care is _____?

a. Appropriateness
b. Medical necessity
c. Benchmarking
d. Evidence-based medicine

141. Assume the patient has already met his or her deductible and that the physician is a Medicare participating (PAR) provider. The physician's standard fee for the services provided is $120.00. Medicare's PAR fee is $60.00. How much reimbursement will the physician receive from Medicare?

a. $120.00
b. $ 48.00
c. $ 96.00
d. $ 60.00

142. Currently, which prospective payment system is used to determine the payment to the physician for outpatient surgery performed on a Medicare patient?

a. ASCs
b. RBRVS
c. MS-DRGs
d. APCs

143. When appropriate, under the outpatient PPS, a hospital can use this CPT code in place of, but not in addition to, a code for a medical visit or emergency department service.

a. 35001
b. 99358
c. 50300
d. 99291

144. The following type of hospital is considered excluded when it applies for and receives a waiver from CMS. This means that the hospital does not participate in the inpatient prospective payment system (IPPS).

a. Psychiatric hospital
b. Cancer hospital
c. Rehabilitation hospital
d. Long-term care hospital

145. CMS adjusts the Medicare Severity DRGs and the reimbursement rates every _____?

a. Calendar year beginning January 1
b. Month
c. Quarter
d. Fiscal year beginning October 1

146. How long does the Health Insurance Portability and Accountability Act (HIPAA) require facilities to retain health insurance claims and accounting records?

a. Six years
b. Seven years
c. Ten years
d. Five years

147. Changes in case-mix index (CMI) may be attributed to all of the following factors EXCEPT _____?

a. Changes in services offered.
b. Changes in coding rules.
c. Changes in medical staff composition.
d. Changes in coding productivity.

148. If a participating provider's usual fee for a service is $700.00 and Medicare's allowed amount is $450.00, what amount is written off by the physician?

a. None of it is written off
b. $340.00
c. $391.00
d. $250.00

149. How many major diagnostic categories are there in the MS-DRG system?

a. 2,000
b. 25
c. 80
d. 100

150. The standard claim form used by hospitals to request reimbursement for inpatient and outpatient procedures performed or services provided is called _____?

a. CMS-1600
b. CMS-1500
c. CMS-1491
d. UB-04

RHIT Mock Exam - Answers

Domain 1 - Data Analysis and Management (Answers)

1. a. The needs of the user should alway be the primary concern.

2. c. HAVEN (Home Assessment Validation and Entry) is available on the OASIS website.

3. c. The gross hospital death rate is figured by dividing the total number of discharges by the total number of deaths.

4. b. Problems are always organized in numeric order.

5. a. Uniform Hospital Discharge Data Set is the first resource used.

6. c. Minimum Data Set is considered the minimum amount needed to know about any one person, per Medicare guidelines, to provide appropriate, individualized care to that person.

7. d. Data accountability is not a characteristic of high quality healthcare.

8. d. Calculation is: (500/50) + (500/40) = 22.5 Hours per day

9. b. Census. Do not be fooled into Average daily census which is the mean number of patients.

10. c. A patients complete medical history is not documented in an emergency record.

11. a. Data is factual without giving any meaning to the facts. Information offers meaning and explanation.

12. d. Daily inpatient census.

13. c. Incidence in epidemiology is a measure of the probability of occurrence of a given medical condition in a population within a specified period of time. Although sometimes loosely expressed simply as the number of new cases during some time period, it is better expressed as a proportion or a rate with a denominator.

14. a. Evaluate patterns and trends in patient care.

15. c. Uniform Ambulatory Care Data Sets include patient specific items for outpatient care.

16. c. The math is: (10,000 X 0.07) 200 = 140,000.

17. b. OASIS (Outcome and Assessment Information Set).

18. c. Outcomes.

19. a. HEDIS (Healthcare Effectiveness Data and Information Set).

20. a. Minimum Data Set Version 2.0

21. a. HCPCS. The Healthcare Common Procedure Coding System is a set of health care procedure codes based on the American Medical Association's Current Procedural Terminology (CPT).

22. b. A unit of measure that reflects the services received by one inpatient in a 24-hour period is called an inpatient service day. The number of inpatient service days for a 24-hour period is equal to the daily inpatient census - that is, one service day for each patient treated. The calculation is: [(250+30) - 40] + 2 = 242

PROPERTY OF MEDICAL CODING PRO UNAUTHORIZED DISTRIBUTION PROHIBITED SINGLE COPY LICENSE

23. b. Select a representative set of data elements and track these across the database to identify consistencies and differences.

24. a. Data Sets

25. d. The International Classification of Diseases - 10th Revision - Clinical Modification.

26. c. Abstracting.

27. a. CMS uses the Minimum Data Set for long term care.

28. c. Determine the volume and type of data stored within each database so that the repository of similar data can be developed.

29. b. Data Dictionary.

30. d. Continuity of Care Record.

Domain 2 - Coding (Answers)

31. a. Accuracy and volume.

32. c. D23.11 Other benign neoplasm of skin of right eyelid, including canthus.

33. b. Healthcare Common Procedure Coding System (HCPCS).

34. b. The Civilian Health and Medical Program of the Department of Veterans Affairs (CHAMPVA) is a comprehensive health care program in which the VA shares the cost of covered health care services and supplies with eligible beneficiaries.

35. c. 0S523ZZ, Destruction of Lumbar Vertebral Disc, Percutaneous Approach.

36. d. SNOMED CT is the most comprehensive and precise clinical health terminology product in the world, owned and distributed around the world by The International Health Terminology Standards Development Organization (IHTSDO).

37. b. The correct sequencing is: Congestive heart failure, respiratory failure, ventilator management, intubation.

38. b. Placenta previa is an obstetric complication in which the placenta lies in the uterus and covers all or part of the opening to the cervix.

39. a. The Ambulatory Payment Classifications payment system is based on CPT and HCPCS codes.

40. a. Differentiate between conditions present on admission and conditions that develop during an inpatient admission. As part of the Deficit Reduction Act, CMS now requires hospitals to enter POA indicators on all inpatient acute-care hospital claims.

PROPERTY OF MEDICAL CODING PRO UNAUTHORIZED DISTRIBUTION PROHIBITED SINGLE COPY LICENSE

41. b. A Diagnosis-Related Group (DRG) is a statistical system of classifying any inpatient stay into groups for the purposes of payment. It divides possible diagnoses into more than 20 major body systems and subdivides them into almost 500 groups for the purpose of Medicare reimbursement.

42. c. Query the physician to ask if the patient has septicemia because of the symptomatology.

43. a. Beginning the day the Medicare patient is admitted to the hospital and ending when the patient has not been hospitalized for a period of sixty consecutive days.

44. d. Workers' compensation is a form of insurance providing wage replacement and medical benefits to employees injured in the course of employment in exchange for mandatory relinquishment of the employee's right to sue his or her employer for the tort of negligence.

45. a. Since October 1, 1983, most hospitals have been paid under the hospital inpatient prospective payment system (PPS). However, certain types of specialty hospitals and units were excluded from PPS because the PPS DRG's do not accurately account for the resource costs for the types of patients treated in those facilities. Facilities originally excluded from PPS included rehabilitation, psychiatric, children's, cancer, and long term care hospitals, rehabilitation and psychiatric hospital distinct part units, and hospitals located outside the 50 states and Puerto Rico.

46. d. The hospital outpatient prospective payment system (OPPS) classifies all hospital outpatient services into APCs. HCPCS codes are assigned to APCs by CMS, and these assignments are updated at least annually.

RHIT Practice Exam Bundle 2017   75

47. c. The State Children's Health Insurance Program (SCHIP) is a partnership between the Federal and state governments that provides health coverage to uninsured children whose families earn too much to qualify for Medicaid, but too little to afford private coverage.

48. a. Sequence either the pancreatitis or the noncalculus cholecystitis as the principal diagnosis.

49. b. Fever, cough, shortness of breath

50. c. The International Classification of Diseases for Oncology (ICD-O)3 was published in 2000 and used principally in tumor or cancer registries, for coding the site (topography) and the histology (morphology) of the neoplasm, usually obtained from a pathology report.

51. b. The Diagnostic and Statistical Manual of Mental Disorders, Fifth Edition (DSM-5) is the 2013 update to the American Psychiatric Association's (APA) classification and diagnostic tool. In the United States the DSM serves as a universal authority for psychiatric diagnosis. Treatment recommendations, as well as payment by health care providers, are often determined by DSM classifications, so the appearance of a new version has significant practical importance.

52. a. Hypertension. Pericardia belongs to a class of medications called calcium channel blockers (CCBs) that are used to treat angina (heart pain), high blood pressure, and abnormal heart rhythms.

53. d. The ICD-10 Coordination and Maintenance Committee (C&M) is a Federal interdepartmental committee comprised of representatives from the Centers for Medicare and Medicaid Services (CMS) and the Centers for Disease Control and Prevention's (CDC), and the National Center for Health Statistics (NCHS). The committee is responsible for approving coding changes, developing errata, addenda and other modifications.

54. d. Discounting of procedures.

PROPERTY OF MEDICAL CODING PRO UNAUTHORIZED DISTRIBUTION PROHIBITED SINGLE COPY LICENSE

55. c. Cystourethroscopy, with fulguration (including cryosurgery or laser surgery) and/ or resection of large bladder tumors.

Domain 3 - Compliance (Answers)

56. a. Although a gross description of tissue removed may be mentioned on the operative note or discharge summary, only the pathology report will contain a microscopic description.

57. a. Use of prohibited or "dangerous" abbreviations.

58. b. DEEDS is intended for use by individuals and organizations responsible for maintaining or improving record systems in 24-hour, hospital-based emergency departments. DEEDS is designed to provide uniform specifications for data elements that decision makers may choose to retain, revise, or add to their ED record systems.

59. c. CMS standards. MDS data are reported directly to the Centers for Medicare and Medicaid Services and must conform to agency standards.

60. b. Security training is provided to all levels of staff.

61. b. Medical records must be retained in their original or legally reproduced form for a period of at least 5 years.

62. b. Conduct audit trails to monitor inappropriate access to system information. The other three answers deal with privacy, not internal security.

63. c. Federal Register. CMS publishes both proposed and final rules for the Conditions of Participation for hospitals in the daily Federal Register.

64. a. Master Patient Index (MPI) is an electronic medical database that holds information on every patient registered at a healthcare organization. It may also include data on physicians, other medical staff and facility employees.

65. c. Educate physicians regarding proper documentation policies and standards.

66. a. When a file is removed or "checked out," an outguide is used in its place to alert personnel that the file is being used or has been removed.

67. c. Age of majority plus statute of limitation unless state or federal laws require longer time periods.

68. b. The courts do not have to be notified of the record destruction.

69. c. Missing operative reports. Institutions are given a Type I recommendation when 2% of delinquent records are due to missing history and physicals or operative reports. The remaining choices are incorrect and defined as follows: absence of SOAP format in progress notes = the SOAP format is not a requirement of Joint Commission; missing signatures on progress notes = both signature omissions and discharge summary reports can be captured after discharge, but history and physicals should be on the chart within 24 hours of the patient's admission; missing discharge summaries = both signature omissions and discharge summary reports can be captured after discharge, but history and physicals should be on the chart within 24 hours of the patient's admission.

70. d. A physician index does not have to be retained permanently.

71. a. Required for reimbursement of certain patient groups. The remaining choices are incorrect and explained as follows: required for state licensure in all states = state licensure is required for accreditation but not the reverse; considered unnecessary by most health care facilities = advantages of accreditation are numerous and include financial and legal incentives; conducted in each facility annually = joint Commission conducts unannounced on-site surveys approximately every three years.

72. c. Statutory requirements.

73. b. Achieving meaningful use of EHRs. There are several core objectives for achieving meaningful use. Engaging patients and their families is one.

74. b. The Commission on Cancer (CoC) of the American College of Surgeons (ACoS) requires approved cancer programs to meet or exceed the target rate of 90 percent successful follow-up. SEER cancer registries must meet or exceed 95% successful follow-up. The follow-up rate is calculated on all eligible patients, both living and dead.

75. d. Trauma Registry. The Injury Severity Score (ISS) is an established medical score to assess trauma severity. It correlates with mortality, morbidity and hospitalization time after trauma. It is used to define the term major trauma.

76. b. MDS. OBRA mandates comprehensive functional assessments of long-term care residents using the Minimum Data Set for long-term care.

77. a. Delegated use of computer key by radiology secretary. Written signatures, identifiable initials, unique computer codes, and rubber stamp signatures may all be allowed as legitimate means of authenticating an entry. However, the use of codes and stamped signatures MUST be confined to the owners and they are never to be used by anyone else.

78. b. The presence or absence of such items as preoperative and postoperative. The following choices are incorrect and defined as follows: the quality of follow-up care = represents the clinical care evaluation process rather than the review of quality documentation; whether the severity of illness and/or intensity of service warranted acute level care = this is a function of the utilization review program; whether a postoperative infection occurred and how it was treated = this represents an appropriate job for the infection control officer.

79. b. The facility must match the states statute of limitations period of seven years.

80. c. Use CPOE for medication orders. See all objectives for Stage I of meaningful use on the www.healthit.gov website.

Domain 4 - Information Technologies (Answers)

81. b. Relational databases store data in predefined tables similar to a spreadsheet and are often used in healthcare applications.

82. d. Computer station that promotes the healthcare organization's services.

83. c. Pharmacy information system uses standard order sets and clinical decision support to assist the providers. Once the provider's orders are checked by the CDS and the physician signs off the orders are routed to their destination.

84. a. Client/ server allows for the sharing of a database, printers, disc space, etc. across a network.

85. d. All of the above.

86. b. An Electronic Document Management System (EDMS) is a collection of technologies that work together to provide a comprehensive solution for managing the creation, capture, indexing, storage, retrieval, and disposition of records and information assets of the organization.

87. a. A transaction process system (TPS) is an information processing system for business transactions involving the collection, modification and retrieval of all transaction data.

88. c. Database management system. One of the main functions of the DBMS is security to prevent unauthorized access.

89. d. Planning is used to adopt new IS technology and identifying and assigning priorities and various upgrades.

90. c. Assembly. This function is replaced by record preparation and document scanning.

91. c. Actual patient data to ensure accuracy.

92. a. Combine information from any system within the organization. Interoperability allows information to be shared from one computer system to another.

93. c. Identity matching algorithm. HIE organizations utilize probability equations to identify patients.

94. a. Clinical Data Warehouse (CDW) is a real time database that consolidates data from a variety of clinical sources to present a unified view of a single patient.

95. a. The Certification Commission for Healthcare Information Technology (CCHIT) is an independent, not-for-profit group that certifies electronic health records (EHR) and networks for health information exchange (HIE) in the United States.

96. a. Cryptography is for data security. The other answers are for systems security.

97. c. Application safeguards such as password management are contained within the application software.

98. a. EHR's are based on the use of a clinical data repository. A CDR is a database that manages data from different source systems in the hospital or provider settings, they can also store and make accessible paper document images and clinical images such as those from PACS.

99. c. HL7 is an ANSI-accredited standards developing organization that provides comprehensive standards for exchange, integration, sharing and retrieving of electronic health information among hospital systems and provider systems.

RHIT Practice Exam Bundle 2017   83

100. a. Help manage work tasks. Workflow support has also been added to Electronic Document Management Systems and these functions can work in sequence or simultaneously.

PROPERTY OF MEDICAL CODING PRO UNAUTHORIZED DISTRIBUTION PROHIBITED SINGLE COPY LICENSE

Domain 5 - Quality (Answers)

101. a. Root cause analysis (RCA) is a method of problem solving used for identifying the root causes of faults or problems.

102. a. Quantitative analysis refers to economic, business or financial analysis that aims to understand or predict behavior or events through the use of mathematical measurements and calculations, statistical modeling and research.

103. a. Define what is to be studied and accomplished by instituting benchmarks. Benchmarking is comparing one's business processes and performance metrics to industry bests and best practices from other companies.

104. b. Patient history of inhaled food, liquid or oil.

105. a. Deemed status. Health care organizations that achieve accreditation through a Joint Commission deemed status survey are determined to meet or exceed Medicare and Medicaid requirements.

106. d. Arrive at the desired outcomes.

107. c. Conduct medical peer review to identify patterns of care.

108. b. Operational planning. Operational planning is the process of planning strategic goals and objectives to tactical goals and objectives.

109. a. HEDIS. The Healthcare Effectiveness Data and Information Set (HEDIS) is a tool used by more than 90 percent of America's health plans to measure performance on important dimensions of care and service. Altogether, HEDIS consists of 81 measures across 5 domains of care.

110. d. A continuous cycle of improvement.

RHIT Practice Exam Bundle 2017   85

111. c. Both system and patient tracers.

112. b. Care planning at the time of admission.

113. c. Peer review.

114. b. Benchmark. Benchmarking is comparing one's business processes and performance metrics to industry bests and best practices from other companies.

115. d. Outcome indicator. Outcome indicators are measures that describe how well we are achieving our outcomes. They help us know whether things are changing in the way we intended.

116. a. Determination of the quickest solution.

117. c. Quality Improvement. They tell us how well something is being done or not done, variances from our standard performance.

118. c. Providers.

119. a. Addressing employee resistance to change.

120. b. Where very small deviations can have a significant impact. Six Sigma is a disciplined, data-driven approach and methodology for eliminating defects in any process, from manufacturing to transactional and from product to service.

PROPERTY OF MEDICAL CODING PRO UNAUTHORIZED DISTRIBUTION PROHIBITED SINGLE COPY LICENSE

Domain 6 - Legal (Answers)

121. b. ARRA mandates that a CE must comply with a requested restriction unless it meets one of the exceptions.

122. d. Workforce clearance procedure.

123. c. The patient is an exception to the minimum necessary rule so process the request as written.

124. a. Under the OSH Act, employers are responsible for providing a safe and healthful workplace. Occupational Safety and Health Administration's (OSHA) mission is to assure safe and healthful workplaces by setting and enforcing standards, and by providing training, outreach, education and assistance.

125. b. The facility has 30 days to comply with the request.

126. a. Develop a plan for reporting privacy complaints. The other options would be the responsibility of the Chief Security Officer.

127. a. Bona fide occupational qualification. Title VII permits you to discriminate on the basis of "religion, sex, or national origin in those instances where religion, sex, or national origin is a bona fide occupational qualification reasonably necessary to the normal operation of the particular business or enterprise."

128. d. Statutes of limitations. A statute of limitation is a law which forbids prosecutors from charging someone with a crime that was committed more than a specified number of years ago. The general purpose of statutes of limitation is to make sure convictions occur only upon evidence (physical or eyewitness) that has not deteriorated with time.

129. a. Physical/ workstation security.

PROPERTY OF MEDICAL CODING PRO UNAUTHORIZED DISTRIBUTION PROHIBITED SINGLE COPY LICENSE

130. c. Incidental disclosures occur when people see or hear protected health information (PHI) when they do not have a "need to know" that specific information. The Privacy Rule permits certain incidental disclosures that occur as a by-product of another permissible or required use of the information.

131. a. Follow the incident response procedure. An Incident response is an organized approach to addressing and managing the aftermath of a security breach or attack (also known as an incident).

132. a. The Institutional Review Board deals with the ethical treatment of human research subjects. The Ethics Committee covers a wide range of issues.

133. b. The thickness of the records.

134. b. When federal and state laws conflict, valid federal laws supersede state laws.

135. d. Remove any information that might prove detrimental to the hospital or physician.

RHIT Practice Exam Bundle 2017   88

Domain 7 - Revenue Cycle (Answers)

136. a. Medical visits are not packaged under Medicare OPP.

137. d. If a physician is a participating physician who accepts assignment, he will receive the lesser of "the total charges" or "the PAR Medicare fee schedule amount." In this case, the Medicare fee schedule amount is less; therefore, the total received by the physician is $200.00.

138. d. The software program is called a grouper.

139. b. Cost accounting is a process of collecting, recording, classifying, analyzing, summarizing, allocating and evaluating various alternative courses of action & control of costs. Its goal is to advise the management on the most appropriate course of action based on the cost efficiency and capability.

140. b. Medical necessity is a United States legal doctrine, related to activities which may be justified as reasonable, necessary, and/or appropriate, based on evidence-based clinical standards of care.

141. b.$ 48.00. If the physician is a participating physician (PAR) who accepts the assignment, he will receive the lesser of the "total charges" or the "PAR amount" (on the Medicare Physician Fee Schedule). Since the PAR amount is lower, the physician collects 80% of the PAR amount ($60.00) x .80 =$48.00, from Medicare. The remaining 20% ($60.00 x .20 = $12.00) of the PAR amount is paid by the patient to the physician. Therefore, the physician will receive $48.00 directly from Medicare.

142. b. RBRVS. Resource Based Relative Value Scale (RBRVS) is a schema used to determine how much money medical providers should be paid. It is partially used by Medicare in the United States and by nearly all health maintenance organizations (HMOs).

PROPERTY OF MEDICAL CODING PRO UNAUTHORIZED DISTRIBUTION PROHIBITED SINGLE COPY LICENSE

143. d. CPT Code 99291 (critical care). When a patient meets the definition of critical care, the hospital must use CPT Code 99291 to bill for outpatient encounters in which critical care services are furnished. This code is used instead of another E&M code.

144. b. Cancer hospital. Cancer hospitals can apply for and receive waivers from the Centers for Medicare and Medicaid Services (CMS) and are therefore excluded from the inpatient prospective payment system (MS-DRGs). Rehabilitation hospitals are reimbursed under the Inpatient Rehabilitation Prospective Payment System (IRF PPS). Long-term care hospitals are reimbursed under the Long-Term Care Hospital Prospective Payment System (LTCH PPS). Skilled nursing facilities are reimbursed under the Skilled Nursing Facility Prospective Payment System (SNF PPS).

145. d. Fiscal year beginning October 1.

146. a. Six years unless state law specifies a longer period.

147. d. Changes in coding productivity. Coding productivity will not directly affect CMI. Inaccuracy or poor coding quality can affect CMI.

148. d. $250. The participating physician agrees to accept Medicare's fee as payment in full. The physician would write off the difference between $700.00 and $450.00, which is 250.00.

149. There are 25 major diagnostic categories in the MS-DRG system.

150. d. The standard claim form is a UB-04.

Page Left Blank Intentionally.

Scoring Sheet 4

1) A B C D
2) A B C D
3) A B C D
4) A B C D
5) A B C D
6) A B C D
7) A B C D
8) A B C D
9) A B C D
10) A B C D
11) A B C D
12) A B C D
13) A B C D
14) A B C D
15) A B C D
16) A B C D
17) A B C D
18) A B C D
19) A B C D
20) A B C D
21) A B C D
22) A B C D
23) A B C D
24) A B C D
25) A B C D

26) A B C D
27) A B C D
28) A B C D
29) A B C D
30) A B C D
31) A B C D
32) A B C D
33) A B C D
34) A B C D
35) A B C D
36) A B C D
37) A B C D
38) A B C D
39) A B C D
40) A B C D
41) A B C D
42) A B C D
43) A B C D
44) A B C D
45) A B C D
46) A B C D
47) A B C D
48) A B C D
49) A B C D
50) A B C D
51) A B C D
52) A B C D
53) A B C D

54) A B C D
55) A B C D
56) A B C D
57) A B C D
58) A B C D
59) A B C D
60) A B C D
61) A B C D
62) A B C D
63) A B C D
64) A B C D
65) A B C D
66) A B C D
67) A B C D
68) A B C D
69) A B C D
70) A B C D
71) A B C D
72) A B C D
73) A B C D
74) A B C D
75) A B C D
76) A B C D
77) A B C D
78) A B C D
79) A B C D
80) A B C D
81) A B C D

RHIT Practice Exam Bundle 2017   98

82) A B C D   109) A B C D   136) A B C D
83) A B C D   110) A B C D   137) A B C D
84) A B C D   111) A B C D   138) A B C D
85) A B C D   112) A B C D   139) A B C D
86) A B C D   113) A B C D   140) A B C D
87) A B C D   114) A B C D   141) A B C D
88) A B C D   115) A B C D   142) A B C D
89) A B C D   116) A B C D   143) A B C D
90) A B C D   117) A B C D   144) A B C D
91) A B C D   118) A B C D   145) A B C D
92) A B C D   119) A B C D   146) A B C D
93) A B C D   120) A B C D   147) A B C D
94) A B C D   121) A B C D   148) A B C D
95) A B C D   122) A B C D   149) A B C D
96) A B C D   123) A B C D   150) A B C D
97) A B C D   124) A B C D
98) A B C D   125) A B C D   XXXXXXXXXXXXXXX
99) A B C D   126) A B C D   XXXXXXXXXXXXXXX
100) A B C D   127) A B C D   XXXXXXXXXXXXXXX
101) A B C D   128) A B C D   XXXXXXXXXXXXXXX
102) A B C D   129) A B C D
103) A B C D   130) A B C D
104) A B C D   131) A B C D
105) A B C D   132) A B C D
106) A B C D   133) A B C D
107) A B C D   134) A B C D
108) A B C D   135) A B C D

PROPERTY OF MEDICAL CODING PRO UNAUTHORIZED DISTRIBUTION PROHIBITED SINGLE COPY LICENSE

Scoring Sheet 5

1)	A	B	C	D	26)	A	B	C	D	54)	A	B	C	D
2)	A	B	C	D	27)	A	B	C	D	55)	A	B	C	D
3)	A	B	C	D	28)	A	B	C	D	56)	A	B	C	D
4)	A	B	C	D	29)	A	B	C	D	57)	A	B	C	D
5)	A	B	C	D	30)	A	B	C	D	58)	A	B	C	D
6)	A	B	C	D	31)	A	B	C	D	59)	A	B	C	D
7)	A	B	C	D	32)	A	B	C	D	60)	A	B	C	D
8)	A	B	C	D	33)	A	B	C	D	61)	A	B	C	D
9)	A	B	C	D	34)	A	B	C	D	62)	A	B	C	D
10)	A	B	C	D	35)	A	B	C	D	63)	A	B	C	D
11)	A	B	C	D	36)	A	B	C	D	64)	A	B	C	D
12)	A	B	C	D	37)	A	B	C	D	65)	A	B	C	D
13)	A	B	C	D	38)	A	B	C	D	66)	A	B	C	D
14)	A	B	C	D	39)	A	B	C	D	67)	A	B	C	D
15)	A	B	C	D	40)	A	B	C	D	68)	A	B	C	D
16)	A	B	C	D	41)	A	B	C	D	69)	A	B	C	D
17)	A	B	C	D	42)	A	B	C	D	70)	A	B	C	D
18)	A	B	C	D	43)	A	B	C	D	71)	A	B	C	D
19)	A	B	C	D	44)	A	B	C	D	72)	A	B	C	D
20)	A	B	C	D	45)	A	B	C	D	73)	A	B	C	D
21)	A	B	C	D	46)	A	B	C	D	74)	A	B	C	D
22)	A	B	C	D	47)	A	B	C	D	75)	A	B	C	D
23)	A	B	C	D	48)	A	B	C	D	76)	A	B	C	D
24)	A	B	C	D	49)	A	B	C	D	77)	A	B	C	D
25)	A	B	C	D	50)	A	B	C	D	78)	A	B	C	D
					51)	A	B	C	D	79)	A	B	C	D
					52)	A	B	C	D	80)	A	B	C	D
					53)	A	B	C	D	81)	A	B	C	D

PROPERTY OF MEDICAL CODING PRO UNAUTHORIZED DISTRIBUTION PROHIBITED SINGLE COPY LICENSE

82)	A	B	C	D	109)	A	B	C	D	136)	A	B	C	D
83)	A	B	C	D	110)	A	B	C	D	137)	A	B	C	D
84)	A	B	C	D	111)	A	B	C	D	138)	A	B	C	D
85)	A	B	C	D	112)	A	B	C	D	139)	A	B	C	D
86)	A	B	C	D	113)	A	B	C	D	140)	A	B	C	D
87)	A	B	C	D	114)	A	B	C	D	141)	A	B	C	D
88)	A	B	C	D	115)	A	B	C	D	142)	A	B	C	D
89)	A	B	C	D	116)	A	B	C	D	143)	A	B	C	D
90)	A	B	C	D	117)	A	B	C	D	144)	A	B	C	D
91)	A	B	C	D	118)	A	B	C	D	145)	A	B	C	D
92)	A	B	C	D	119)	A	B	C	D	146)	A	B	C	D
93)	A	B	C	D	120)	A	B	C	D	147)	A	B	C	D
94)	A	B	C	D	121)	A	B	C	D	148)	A	B	C	D
95)	A	B	C	D	122)	A	B	C	D	149)	A	B	C	D
96)	A	B	C	D	123)	A	B	C	D	150)	A	B	C	D
97)	A	B	C	D	124)	A	B	C	D
98)	A	B	C	D	125)	A	B	C	D
99)	A	B	C	D	126)	A	B	C	D
100)	A	B	C	D	127)	A	B	C	D
101)	A	B	C	D	128)	A	B	C	D
102)	A	B	C	D	129)	A	B	C	D
103)	A	B	C	D	130)	A	B	C	D
104)	A	B	C	D	131)	A	B	C	D
105)	A	B	C	D	132)	A	B	C	D
106)	A	B	C	D	133)	A	B	C	D
107)	A	B	C	D	134)	A	B	C	D
108)	A	B	C	D	135)	A	B	C	D

XXXXXXXXXXXXXX
XXXXXXXXXXXXXX
XXXXXXXXXXXXXX
XXXXXXXXXXXXXX

Scoring Sheet 6

1)   A   B   C   D
2)   A   B   C   D
3)   A   B   C   D
4)   A   B   C   D
5)   A   B   C   D
6)   A   B   C   D
7)   A   B   C   D
8)   A   B   C   D
9)   A   B   C   D
10)   A   B   C   D
11)   A   B   C   D
12)   A   B   C   D
13)   A   B   C   D
14)   A   B   C   D
15)   A   B   C   D
16)   A   B   C   D
17)   A   B   C   D
18)   A   B   C   D
19)   A   B   C   D
20)   A   B   C   D
21)   A   B   C   D
22)   A   B   C   D
23)   A   B   C   D
24)   A   B   C   D
25)   A   B   C   D

26)   A   B   C   D
27)   A   B   C   D
28)   A   B   C   D
29)   A   B   C   D
30)   A   B   C   D
31)   A   B   C   D
32)   A   B   C   D
33)   A   B   C   D
34)   A   B   C   D
35)   A   B   C   D
36)   A   B   C   D
37)   A   B   C   D
38)   A   B   C   D
39)   A   B   C   D
40)   A   B   C   D
41)   A   B   C   D
42)   A   B   C   D
43)   A   B   C   D
44)   A   B   C   D
45)   A   B   C   D
46)   A   B   C   D
47)   A   B   C   D
48)   A   B   C   D
49)   A   B   C   D
50)   A   B   C   D
51)   A   B   C   D
52)   A   B   C   D
53)   A   B   C   D

54)   A   B   C   D
55)   A   B   C   D
56)   A   B   C   D
57)   A   B   C   D
58)   A   B   C   D
59)   A   B   C   D
60)   A   B   C   D
61)   A   B   C   D
62)   A   B   C   D
63)   A   B   C   D
64)   A   B   C   D
65)   A   B   C   D
66)   A   B   C   D
67)   A   B   C   D
68)   A   B   C   D
69)   A   B   C   D
70)   A   B   C   D
71)   A   B   C   D
72)   A   B   C   D
73)   A   B   C   D
74)   A   B   C   D
75)   A   B   C   D
76)   A   B   C   D
77)   A   B   C   D
78)   A   B   C   D
79)   A   B   C   D
80)   A   B   C   D
81)   A   B   C   D

82)	A	B	C	D		109)	A	B	C	D		136)	A	B	C	D
83)	A	B	C	D		110)	A	B	C	D		137)	A	B	C	D
84)	A	B	C	D		111)	A	B	C	D		138)	A	B	C	D
85)	A	B	C	D		112)	A	B	C	D		139)	A	B	C	D
86)	A	B	C	D		113)	A	B	C	D		140)	A	B	C	D
87)	A	B	C	D		114)	A	B	C	D		141)	A	B	C	D
88)	A	B	C	D		115)	A	B	C	D		142)	A	B	C	D
89)	A	B	C	D		116)	A	B	C	D		143)	A	B	C	D
90)	A	B	C	D		117)	A	B	C	D		144)	A	B	C	D
91)	A	B	C	D		118)	A	B	C	D		145)	A	B	C	D
92)	A	B	C	D		119)	A	B	C	D		146)	A	B	C	D
93)	A	B	C	D		120)	A	B	C	D		147)	A	B	C	D
94)	A	B	C	D		121)	A	B	C	D		148)	A	B	C	D
95)	A	B	C	D		122)	A	B	C	D		149)	A	B	C	D
96)	A	B	C	D		123)	A	B	C	D		150)	A	B	C	D
97)	A	B	C	D		124)	A	B	C	D						
98)	A	B	C	D		125)	A	B	C	D		XXXXXXXXXXXXXXX				
99)	A	B	C	D		126)	A	B	C	D		XXXXXXXXXXXXXXX				
100)	A	B	C	D		127)	A	B	C	D		XXXXXXXXXXXXXXX				
101)	A	B	C	D		128)	A	B	C	D		XXXXXXXXXXXXXXX				
102)	A	B	C	D		129)	A	B	C	D						
103)	A	B	C	D		130)	A	B	C	D						
104)	A	B	C	D		131)	A	B	C	D						
105)	A	B	C	D		132)	A	B	C	D						
106)	A	B	C	D		133)	A	B	C	D						
107)	A	B	C	D		134)	A	B	C	D						
108)	A	B	C	D		135)	A	B	C	D						

Scoring Sheet 7

1) A B C D
2) A B C D
3) A B C D
4) A B C D
5) A B C D
6) A B C D
7) A B C D
8) A B C D
9) A B C D
10) A B C D
11) A B C D
12) A B C D
13) A B C D
14) A B C D
15) A B C D
16) A B C D
17) A B C D
18) A B C D
19) A B C D
20) A B C D
21) A B C D
22) A B C D
23) A B C D
24) A B C D
25) A B C D

26) A B C D
27) A B C D
28) A B C D
29) A B C D
30) A B C D
31) A B C D
32) A B C D
33) A B C D
34) A B C D
35) A B C D
36) A B C D
37) A B C D
38) A B C D
39) A B C D
40) A B C D
41) A B C D
42) A B C D
43) A B C D
44) A B C D
45) A B C D
46) A B C D
47) A B C D
48) A B C D
49) A B C D
50) A B C D
51) A B C D
52) A B C D
53) A B C D

54) A B C D
55) A B C D
56) A B C D
57) A B C D
58) A B C D
59) A B C D
60) A B C D
61) A B C D
62) A B C D
63) A B C D
64) A B C D
65) A B C D
66) A B C D
67) A B C D
68) A B C D
69) A B C D
70) A B C D
71) A B C D
72) A B C D
73) A B C D
74) A B C D
75) A B C D
76) A B C D
77) A B C D
78) A B C D
79) A B C D
80) A B C D
81) A B C D

82)	A	B	C	D	109)	A	B	C	D	136)	A	B	C	D
83)	A	B	C	D	110)	A	B	C	D	137)	A	B	C	D
84)	A	B	C	D	111)	A	B	C	D	138)	A	B	C	D
85)	A	B	C	D	112)	A	B	C	D	139)	A	B	C	D
86)	A	B	C	D	113)	A	B	C	D	140)	A	B	C	D
87)	A	B	C	D	114)	A	B	C	D	141)	A	B	C	D
88)	A	B	C	D	115)	A	B	C	D	142)	A	B	C	D
89)	A	B	C	D	116)	A	B	C	D	143)	A	B	C	D
90)	A	B	C	D	117)	A	B	C	D	144)	A	B	C	D
91)	A	B	C	D	118)	A	B	C	D	145)	A	B	C	D
92)	A	B	C	D	119)	A	B	C	D	146)	A	B	C	D
93)	A	B	C	D	120)	A	B	C	D	147)	A	B	C	D
94)	A	B	C	D	121)	A	B	C	D	148)	A	B	C	D
95)	A	B	C	D	122)	A	B	C	D	149)	A	B	C	D
96)	A	B	C	D	123)	A	B	C	D	150)	A	B	C	D
97)	A	B	C	D	124)	A	B	C	D					
98)	A	B	C	D	125)	A	B	C	D					
99)	A	B	C	D	126)	A	B	C	D					
100)	A	B	C	D	127)	A	B	C	D					
101)	A	B	C	D	128)	A	B	C	D					
102)	A	B	C	D	129)	A	B	C	D					
103)	A	B	C	D	130)	A	B	C	D					
104)	A	B	C	D	131)	A	B	C	D					
105)	A	B	C	D	132)	A	B	C	D					
106)	A	B	C	D	133)	A	B	C	D					
107)	A	B	C	D	134)	A	B	C	D					
108)	A	B	C	D	135)	A	B	C	D					

XXXXXXXXXXXXXX
XXXXXXXXXXXXXX
XXXXXXXXXXXXXX
XXXXXXXXXXXXXX

Scoring Sheet 8

1)	A	B	C	D
2)	A	B	C	D
3)	A	B	C	D
4)	A	B	C	D
5)	A	B	C	D
6)	A	B	C	D
7)	A	B	C	D
8)	A	B	C	D
9)	A	B	C	D
10)	A	B	C	D
11)	A	B	C	D
12)	A	B	C	D
13)	A	B	C	D
14)	A	B	C	D
15)	A	B	C	D
16)	A	B	C	D
17)	A	B	C	D
18)	A	B	C	D
19)	A	B	C	D
20)	A	B	C	D
21)	A	B	C	D
22)	A	B	C	D
23)	A	B	C	D
24)	A	B	C	D
25)	A	B	C	D
26)	A	B	C	D
27)	A	B	C	D
28)	A	B	C	D
29)	A	B	C	D
30)	A	B	C	D
31)	A	B	C	D
32)	A	B	C	D
33)	A	B	C	D
34)	A	B	C	D
35)	A	B	C	D
36)	A	B	C	D
37)	A	B	C	D
38)	A	B	C	D
39)	A	B	C	D
40)	A	B	C	D
41)	A	B	C	D
42)	A	B	C	D
43)	A	B	C	D
44)	A	B	C	D
45)	A	B	C	D
46)	A	B	C	D
47)	A	B	C	D
48)	A	B	C	D
49)	A	B	C	D
50)	A	B	C	D
51)	A	B	C	D
52)	A	B	C	D
53)	A	B	C	D
54)	A	B	C	D
55)	A	B	C	D
56)	A	B	C	D
57)	A	B	C	D
58)	A	B	C	D
59)	A	B	C	D
60)	A	B	C	D
61)	A	B	C	D
62)	A	B	C	D
63)	A	B	C	D
64)	A	B	C	D
65)	A	B	C	D
66)	A	B	C	D
67)	A	B	C	D
68)	A	B	C	D
69)	A	B	C	D
70)	A	B	C	D
71)	A	B	C	D
72)	A	B	C	D
73)	A	B	C	D
74)	A	B	C	D
75)	A	B	C	D
76)	A	B	C	D
77)	A	B	C	D
78)	A	B	C	D
79)	A	B	C	D
80)	A	B	C	D
81)	A	B	C	D

PROPERTY OF MEDICAL CODING PRO UNAUTHORIZED DISTRIBUTION PROHIBITED SINGLE COPY LICENSE

82)	A	B	C	D	109)	A	B	C	D	136)	A	B	C	D
83)	A	B	C	D	110)	A	B	C	D	137)	A	B	C	D
84)	A	B	C	D	111)	A	B	C	D	138)	A	B	C	D
85)	A	B	C	D	112)	A	B	C	D	139)	A	B	C	D
86)	A	B	C	D	113)	A	B	C	D	140)	A	B	C	D
87)	A	B	C	D	114)	A	B	C	D	141)	A	B	C	D
88)	A	B	C	D	115)	A	B	C	D	142)	A	B	C	D
89)	A	B	C	D	116)	A	B	C	D	143)	A	B	C	D
90)	A	B	C	D	117)	A	B	C	D	144)	A	B	C	D
91)	A	B	C	D	118)	A	B	C	D	145)	A	B	C	D
92)	A	B	C	D	119)	A	B	C	D	146)	A	B	C	D
93)	A	B	C	D	120)	A	B	C	D	147)	A	B	C	D
94)	A	B	C	D	121)	A	B	C	D	148)	A	B	C	D
95)	A	B	C	D	122)	A	B	C	D	149)	A	B	C	D
96)	A	B	C	D	123)	A	B	C	D	150)	A	B	C	D
97)	A	B	C	D	124)	A	B	C	D					
98)	A	B	C	D	125)	A	B	C	D	XXXXXXXXXXXXXX				
99)	A	B	C	D	126)	A	B	C	D	XXXXXXXXXXXXXX				
100)	A	B	C	D	127)	A	B	C	D	XXXXXXXXXXXXXX				
101)	A	B	C	D	128)	A	B	C	D	XXXXXXXXXXXXXX				
102)	A	B	C	D	129)	A	B	C	D					
103)	A	B	C	D	130)	A	B	C	D					
104)	A	B	C	D	131)	A	B	C	D					
105)	A	B	C	D	132)	A	B	C	D					
106)	A	B	C	D	133)	A	B	C	D					
107)	A	B	C	D	134)	A	B	C	D					
108)	A	B	C	D	135)	A	B	C	D					

PROPERTY OF MEDICAL CODING PRO UNAUTHORIZED DISTRIBUTION PROHIBITED SINGLE COPY LICENSE

Scoring Sheet 9

1)	A	B	C	D	26)	A	B	C	D	54)	A	B	C	D

1) A B C D
2) A B C D
3) A B C D
4) A B C D
5) A B C D
6) A B C D
7) A B C D
8) A B C D
9) A B C D
10) A B C D
11) A B C D
12) A B C D
13) A B C D
14) A B C D
15) A B C D
16) A B C D
17) A B C D
18) A B C D
19) A B C D
20) A B C D
21) A B C D
22) A B C D
23) A B C D
24) A B C D
25) A B C D

26) A B C D
27) A B C D
28) A B C D
29) A B C D
30) A B C D
31) A B C D
32) A B C D
33) A B C D
34) A B C D
35) A B C D
36) A B C D
37) A B C D
38) A B C D
39) A B C D
40) A B C D
41) A B C D
42) A B C D
43) A B C D
44) A B C D
45) A B C D
46) A B C D
47) A B C D
48) A B C D
49) A B C D
50) A B C D
51) A B C D
52) A B C D
53) A B C D

54) A B C D
55) A B C D
56) A B C D
57) A B C D
58) A B C D
59) A B C D
60) A B C D
61) A B C D
62) A B C D
63) A B C D
64) A B C D
65) A B C D
66) A B C D
67) A B C D
68) A B C D
69) A B C D
70) A B C D
71) A B C D
72) A B C D
73) A B C D
74) A B C D
75) A B C D
76) A B C D
77) A B C D
78) A B C D
79) A B C D
80) A B C D
81) A B C D

82)	A	B	C	D	109)	A	B	C	D	136)	A	B	C	D
83)	A	B	C	D	110)	A	B	C	D	137)	A	B	C	D
84)	A	B	C	D	111)	A	B	C	D	138)	A	B	C	D
85)	A	B	C	D	112)	A	B	C	D	139)	A	B	C	D
86)	A	B	C	D	113)	A	B	C	D	140)	A	B	C	D
87)	A	B	C	D	114)	A	B	C	D	141)	A	B	C	D
88)	A	B	C	D	115)	A	B	C	D	142)	A	B	C	D
89)	A	B	C	D	116)	A	B	C	D	143)	A	B	C	D
90)	A	B	C	D	117)	A	B	C	D	144)	A	B	C	D
91)	A	B	C	D	118)	A	B	C	D	145)	A	B	C	D
92)	A	B	C	D	119)	A	B	C	D	146)	A	B	C	D
93)	A	B	C	D	120)	A	B	C	D	147)	A	B	C	D
94)	A	B	C	D	121)	A	B	C	D	148)	A	B	C	D
95)	A	B	C	D	122)	A	B	C	D	149)	A	B	C	D
96)	A	B	C	D	123)	A	B	C	D	150)	A	B	C	D
97)	A	B	C	D	124)	A	B	C	D					
98)	A	B	C	D	125)	A	B	C	D					
99)	A	B	C	D	126)	A	B	C	D					
100)	A	B	C	D	127)	A	B	C	D					
101)	A	B	C	D	128)	A	B	C	D					
102)	A	B	C	D	129)	A	B	C	D					
103)	A	B	C	D	130)	A	B	C	D					
104)	A	B	C	D	131)	A	B	C	D					
105)	A	B	C	D	132)	A	B	C	D					
106)	A	B	C	D	133)	A	B	C	D					
107)	A	B	C	D	134)	A	B	C	D					
108)	A	B	C	D	135)	A	B	C	D					

XXXXXXXXXXXXXX
XXXXXXXXXXXXXX
XXXXXXXXXXXXXX
XXXXXXXXXXXXXX

Scoring Sheet 10

1) A B C D
2) A B C D
3) A B C D
4) A B C D
5) A B C D
6) A B C D
7) A B C D
8) A B C D
9) A B C D
10) A B C D
11) A B C D
12) A B C D
13) A B C D
14) A B C D
15) A B C D
16) A B C D
17) A B C D
18) A B C D
19) A B C D
20) A B C D
21) A B C D
22) A B C D
23) A B C D
24) A B C D
25) A B C D

26) A B C D
27) A B C D
28) A B C D
29) A B C D
30) A B C D
31) A B C D
32) A B C D
33) A B C D
34) A B C D
35) A B C D
36) A B C D
37) A B C D
38) A B C D
39) A B C D
40) A B C D
41) A B C D
42) A B C D
43) A B C D
44) A B C D
45) A B C D
46) A B C D
47) A B C D
48) A B C D
49) A B C D
50) A B C D
51) A B C D
52) A B C D
53) A B C D

54) A B C D
55) A B C D
56) A B C D
57) A B C D
58) A B C D
59) A B C D
60) A B C D
61) A B C D
62) A B C D
63) A B C D
64) A B C D
65) A B C D
66) A B C D
67) A B C D
68) A B C D
69) A B C D
70) A B C D
71) A B C D
72) A B C D
73) A B C D
74) A B C D
75) A B C D
76) A B C D
77) A B C D
78) A B C D
79) A B C D
80) A B C D
81) A B C D

RHIT Practice Exam Bundle 2017

82)	A	B	C	D	109)	A	B	C	D	136)	A	B	C	D
83)	A	B	C	D	110)	A	B	C	D	137)	A	B	C	D
84)	A	B	C	D	111)	A	B	C	D	138)	A	B	C	D
85)	A	B	C	D	112)	A	B	C	D	139)	A	B	C	D
86)	A	B	C	D	113)	A	B	C	D	140)	A	B	C	D
87)	A	B	C	D	114)	A	B	C	D	141)	A	B	C	D
88)	A	B	C	D	115)	A	B	C	D	142)	A	B	C	D
89)	A	B	C	D	116)	A	B	C	D	143)	A	B	C	D
90)	A	B	C	D	117)	A	B	C	D	144)	A	B	C	D
91)	A	B	C	D	118)	A	B	C	D	145)	A	B	C	D
92)	A	B	C	D	119)	A	B	C	D	146)	A	B	C	D
93)	A	B	C	D	120)	A	B	C	D	147)	A	B	C	D
94)	A	B	C	D	121)	A	B	C	D	148)	A	B	C	D
95)	A	B	C	D	122)	A	B	C	D	149)	A	B	C	D
96)	A	B	C	D	123)	A	B	C	D	150)	A	B	C	D
97)	A	B	C	D	124)	A	B	C	D					
98)	A	B	C	D	125)	A	B	C	D					
99)	A	B	C	D	126)	A	B	C	D					
100)	A	B	C	D	127)	A	B	C	D					
101)	A	B	C	D	128)	A	B	C	D					
102)	A	B	C	D	129)	A	B	C	D					
103)	A	B	C	D	130)	A	B	C	D					
104)	A	B	C	D	131)	A	B	C	D					
105)	A	B	C	D	132)	A	B	C	D					
106)	A	B	C	D	133)	A	B	C	D					
107)	A	B	C	D	134)	A	B	C	D					
108)	A	B	C	D	135)	A	B	C	D					

XXXXXXXXXXXXXX
XXXXXXXXXXXXXX
XXXXXXXXXXXXXX
XXXXXXXXXXXXXX

PROPERTY OF MEDICAL CODING PRO UNAUTHORIZED DISTRIBUTION PROHIBITED SINGLE COPY LICENSE

Scoring Sheet 11

1) A B C D
2) A B C D
3) A B C D
4) A B C D
5) A B C D
6) A B C D
7) A B C D
8) A B C D
9) A B C D
10) A B C D
11) A B C D
12) A B C D
13) A B C D
14) A B C D
15) A B C D
16) A B C D
17) A B C D
18) A B C D
19) A B C D
20) A B C D
21) A B C D
22) A B C D
23) A B C D
24) A B C D

25) A B C D
26) A B C D
27) A B C D
28) A B C D
29) A B C D
30) A B C D
31) A B C D
32) A B C D
33) A B C D
34) A B C D
35) A B C D
36) A B C D
37) A B C D
38) A B C D
39) A B C D
40) A B C D
41) A B C D
42) A B C D
43) A B C D
44) A B C D
45) A B C D
46) A B C D
47) A B C D
48) A B C D
49) A B C D
50) A B C D
51) A B C D
52) A B C D

53) A B C D
54) A B C D
55) A B C D
56) A B C D
57) A B C D
58) A B C D
59) A B C D
60) A B C D
61) A B C D
62) A B C D
63) A B C D
64) A B C D
65) A B C D
66) A B C D
67) A B C D
68) A B C D
69) A B C D
70) A B C D
71) A B C D
72) A B C D
73) A B C D
74) A B C D
75) A B C D
76) A B C D
77) A B C D
78) A B C D
79) A B C D
80) A B C D

RHIT Practice Exam Bundle 2017   112

81)	A	B	C	D		108)	A	B	C	D		135)	A	B	C	D
82)	A	B	C	D		109)	A	B	C	D		136)	A	B	C	D
83)	A	B	C	D		110)	A	B	C	D		137)	A	B	C	D
84)	A	B	C	D		111)	A	B	C	D		138)	A	B	C	D
85)	A	B	C	D		112)	A	B	C	D		139)	A	B	C	D
86)	A	B	C	D		113)	A	B	C	D		140)	A	B	C	D
87)	A	B	C	D		114)	A	B	C	D		141)	A	B	C	D
88)	A	B	C	D		115)	A	B	C	D		142)	A	B	C	D
89)	A	B	C	D		116)	A	B	C	D		143)	A	B	C	D
90)	A	B	C	D		117)	A	B	C	D		144)	A	B	C	D
91)	A	B	C	D		118)	A	B	C	D		145)	A	B	C	D
92)	A	B	C	D		119)	A	B	C	D		146)	A	B	C	D
93)	A	B	C	D		120)	A	B	C	D		147)	A	B	C	D
94)	A	B	C	D		121)	A	B	C	D		148)	A	B	C	D
95)	A	B	C	D		122)	A	B	C	D		149)	A	B	C	D
96)	A	B	C	D		123)	A	B	C	D		150)	A	B	C	D
97)	A	B	C	D		124)	A	B	C	D						
98)	A	B	C	D		125)	A	B	C	D		XXXXXXXXXXXXXXX
99)	A	B	C	D		126)	A	B	C	D		XXXXXXXXXXXXXXX
100)	A	B	C	D		127)	A	B	C	D		XXXXXXXXXXXXXXX
101)	A	B	C	D		128)	A	B	C	D		XXXXXXXXXXXXXXX
102)	A	B	C	D		129)	A	B	C	D						
103)	A	B	C	D		130)	A	B	C	D						
104)	A	B	C	D		131)	A	B	C	D						
105)	A	B	C	D		132)	A	B	C	D						
106)	A	B	C	D		133)	A	B	C	D						
107)	A	B	C	D		134)	A	B	C	D						

PROPERTY OF MEDICAL CODING PRO UNAUTHORIZED DISTRIBUTION PROHIBITED SINGLE COPY LICENSE

Scoring Sheet 12

1) A B C D
2) A B C D
3) A B C D
4) A B C D
5) A B C D
6) A B C D
7) A B C D
8) A B C D
9) A B C D
10) A B C D
11) A B C D
12) A B C D
13) A B C D
14) A B C D
15) A B C D
16) A B C D
17) A B C D
18) A B C D
19) A B C D
20) A B C D
21) A B C D
22) A B C D
23) A B C D
24) A B C D
25) A B C D

26) A B C D
27) A B C D
28) A B C D
29) A B C D
30) A B C D
31) A B C D
32) A B C D
33) A B C D
34) A B C D
35) A B C D
36) A B C D
37) A B C D
38) A B C D
39) A B C D
40) A B C D
41) A B C D
42) A B C D
43) A B C D
44) A B C D
45) A B C D
46) A B C D
47) A B C D
48) A B C D
49) A B C D
50) A B C D
51) A B C D
52) A B C D
53) A B C D

54) A B C D
55) A B C D
56) A B C D
57) A B C D
58) A B C D
59) A B C D
60) A B C D
61) A B C D
62) A B C D
63) A B C D
64) A B C D
65) A B C D
66) A B C D
67) A B C D
68) A B C D
69) A B C D
70) A B C D
71) A B C D
72) A B C D
73) A B C D
74) A B C D
75) A B C D
76) A B C D
77) A B C D
78) A B C D
79) A B C D
80) A B C D
81) A B C D

82)	A	B	C	D		109)	A	B	C	D		136)	A	B	C	D

82) A B C D   109) A B C D   136) A B C D
83) A B C D   110) A B C D   137) A B C D
84) A B C D   111) A B C D   138) A B C D
85) A B C D   112) A B C D   139) A B C D
86) A B C D   113) A B C D   140) A B C D
87) A B C D   114) A B C D   141) A B C D
88) A B C D   115) A B C D   142) A B C D
89) A B C D   116) A B C D   143) A B C D
90) A B C D   117) A B C D   144) A B C D
91) A B C D   118) A B C D   145) A B C D
92) A B C D   119) A B C D   146) A B C D
93) A B C D   120) A B C D   147) A B C D
94) A B C D   121) A B C D   148) A B C D
95) A B C D   122) A B C D   149) A B C D
96) A B C D   123) A B C D   150) A B C D
97) A B C D   124) A B C D
98) A B C D   125) A B C D   XXXXXXXXXXXXX
99) A B C D   126) A B C D   XXXXXXXXXXXXX
100) A B C D   127) A B C D   XXXXXXXXXXXXX
101) A B C D   128) A B C D   XXXXXXXXXXXXX
102) A B C D   129) A B C D
103) A B C D   130) A B C D
104) A B C D   131) A B C D
105) A B C D   132) A B C D
106) A B C D   133) A B C D
107) A B C D   134) A B C D
108) A B C D   135) A B C D

Secrets To Reducing Exam Stress

What is Stress

Stress is a normal physical response to events that make you feel threatened or upset your balance in some way, such as situations beyond your control.

The body reacts to these situations with physical, mental, and emotional responses that all merge to create what is known as stress.

When you sense danger or events beyond your control the body's defense mechanisms kick into high gear causing a built in chain reaction of events to occur. This is natural for all of us.

Remember the first time someone reprimanded you for something you had done wrong? Not necessarily a parent or relative, but someone in school or at your place of employment where you felt threatened and began feeling stressed and nervous? That was a natural reaction to a set of circumstances that caused you to feel the effects of stress.

This can be a good thing during an emergency or other event but can also be a bad thing when you are trying to concentrate or think clearly for long periods of time, such as during an exam.

What Causes Stress and Anxiety

Stress is caused by fear, plain and simple. The fear of the unknown. The fear of failing. The fear of being unprepared. The fear of loss. The fear of an uncontrollable situation.

Anything beyond our control can cause fear or a sense of danger and this causes the body to release stress hormones, thus increasing your stress and anxiety level.

There are other factors that cause stress too including family, income, job, friends, life situations and others but the main focus of this book is stress directly attributed to exam preparation and taking an exam.

Once you learn how to reduce and manage stress for an exam you can certainly expand its uses to other areas of your life as well. As a matter of fact, I highly recommend that you do. The facts are clear, the less stress you have in your life the longer you will live and the better quality of life you will have.

What Are The Side Effects Of Stress

When stress is not controlled it can cause a significant amount of problems for people taking an exam. You have likely already experienced some of the side effects of stress including:

• Memory Problems

• Lack of Concentration

• Poor Judgement

• Negative Thoughts

• Headaches

• High Blood Pressure

• Upset Stomach

Each of these side effects can affect your exam preparation efforts and performance. As a matter of fact, in some extreme cases it can cause people to "lock up" and have difficulty even taking an exam. These cases are rare but they do exist. If you suffer from this type of reaction you know all too well how difficult it is to perform under these conditions, let alone excel or perform well enough to earn a passing grade.

So how can you control or minimize the effects of stress and even make it work for you?

Learn to Relax

Setting your mind at ease and learning how to relax can reduce stress dramatically. This is much easier said than done, however, there are different techniques to help you relax and each have there own set of benefits.

There are many different ways to relax your mind and body. Some are more difficult than others. Let's begin with an easy way to reduce even the most sever cases of stress.

Slow Breathing

When you begin to feel the effects of stress your breathing accelerates and your heart rate quickens. This is caused by adrenaline being pumped into your system from the body's reaction to a circumstance or situation.

The first thing you have to do is recognize that you are experiencing stress. After you have done that, the easiest and fastest way to reduce your stress level is to slow your breathing.

If you have ever watched a sporting event you have probably seen top athletes using this method to slow their heart rate, reduce adrenaline flow, relax their muscles, and clear their minds.

This helps them think more clearly, react more rapidly, and perform at a higher level. This is exactly what you want to do.

Top athletes do this when adrenaline is not a good thing and can effect performance.

A good example of this is golf. A golfer relies heavily on muscle memory to produce accurate and consistent golf shots. When adrenaline is introduced into their system, say during the final round of a tournament, it can cause a variation in the distance they hit the ball.

This can make them inconsistent at the very time when they need to be the most consistent.

And at the same time... with the stress level now amped up it can cause a player who normally makes sound decisions to now make questionable ones. This is strikingly similar to an exam situation.

Give this method a try. Take a deep breath and exhale slowly. Repeat this several times until your muscles are totally relaxed and your heart rate slows.

Use this method before studying and prior to and during the exam itself! It will help you think more clearly and be able to recall learned information more rapidly. This technique should be the first thing you do when you start to feel anxious or stressed.

"SOMETIMES WHEN PEOPLE ARE UNDER STRESS THEY HATE TO THINK, AND IT'S THE TIME THEY MOST NEED TO THINK."

PRESIDENT BILL CLINTON

Meditation

Please don't be intimidated by the word "meditation". It is not something to fear, rather something to embrace once you know a little more about it.

Meditation can give your mind a chance to take a much needed break, to "shut down", relax and recharge.

The biggest misconception about meditation is that it is something complex. It isn't. It is simply the process of relaxing your mind and body to give it a much needed break. This is exactly what you need to relieve stress.

Time to Meditate

Meditation does not take that long to do and it can be immensely valuable for your mind, body, and spirit. Scheduling a time to meditate is the best way to make sure it happens on a regular basis.

Set aside ten minutes prior to your scheduled study time each day to meditate. This will get you into the routine of doing it. Also schedule ten to twenty minutes prior to taking an exam to meditate when possible. It will help you relax and open your mind for better memory retention during study time and better information recall during exam time.

Meditation Exercises

Follow these simple steps to enjoy a deeper sense of relaxation.

- Sit in a relaxed position.
- Close your eyes.
- Rest your hands, palms up, on your lap.
- Breathe slowly and slightly deeper than normal.

- Concentrate on your breath coming in and going out.
- Quiet your mind. If you are thinking of something try to release the thought and concentrate on breathing again.
- As you become relaxed repeat a calming word or phrase such as "I feel calm" or "I can achieve", or even "I am the best".
- After ten minutes open your eyes slowly.

This should thoroughly relax you and give you positive thoughts and energy. Now your mind is free to accept new information when studying and ready to recall learned information more rapidly and accurately when taking an exam.

Meditation is nothing more than focused relaxation for the mind and body. Look at it this way. You rest your body six to eight hours per night. Sometimes your mind is resting but not always. So your mind doesn't get as much rest as your body does, just as everything else, it needs rest to be able to perform at a high level.

This is good for daily use, but *ultra* effective prior to exam preparation and before an actual exam.

Set Up A Routine

One of the most important actions you can take to reduce stress and anxiety is set up a study routine.

By setting up a regular study routine you remove the stress of trying to find time everyday to study. Schedule the time in advance. Commit to it and stick to it.

You know what time you have to go to work everyday... right? Why not know what time you are going to study everyday? All good habits are scheduled and repeated. Study time should be no different.

Scheduling

The best time to lay out a schedule is about a month to forty five days prior to an exam when possible. All exams are different but mapping out a consistent plan is essential. This is your way to say "this is important to me".

This will give you enough time to review all the material in a timely manner without cramming it all in at the last minute. This alone will reduce your stress level significantly as well as boost your confidence.

How Often Should You Study

A good study routine should consist of regularly scheduled short periods of uninterrupted and focused study time every day. This will give you time to absorb the information when you are alert and can concentrate fully.

Your study time should <u>not</u> consist of hours upon hours of study time in one day and then no study time for several days. This will wear you down and reduce your ability to retain and recall information.

The last minute "all nighter" is the worst thing you can do! This time should only be for a last minute review of the most difficult material.

Plodding through hundreds of pages of information the night before an exam will only deprive you of sleep you desperately need and dilute any information you have already committed to memory.

You might occasionally "luck out" on an exam this way but keep in mind how much better you could have done had you prepared the right way.

How Long Should You Study

The ideal daily study time is an hour to two hours per day maximum! This will ultimately depend on your work, home, family, or school schedule of course but try to arrange something as close to this as possible.

If you schedule four to five hours or more in one day you are most likely defeating the purpose and wasting your time as your retention will start to decrease in hours three and beyond.

This is specially true if you have other commitments that require your time. Scheduling three or more hours of study time per day can actually add MORE stress to your life and reduce your sleeping time.

Either way this is exactly what you want to avoid at all costs! And I do mean ALL COSTS!

Scheduling time each day will keep you mentally fresh and absorbing good information PLUS it will give you the proper time for other commitments too! The outcome... reduce stressed.

Study With A Buddy

Whenever possible try to study with a buddy. Each person brings a different perspective to the learning process. This is a good way to retain new information because you are more focused on the task at hand when you are with someone else.

Plus, when you commit to study with a buddy the chances are you will actually follow through with your scheduled study time. No one likes to break a promise or commitment.

Commitment

Committing to study with a buddy is kind of like working out. It is hard to get motivated and push yourself to workout daily by yourself. That is just a fact. Only the most disciplined people can do this on their own and even some times they find it a challenge.

When you commit to meet a friend to workout it is much easier to keep your routine and commitment. Even though you may not want to workout that day, you recall the commitment you made to your friend and off you go to follow up on your commitment.

That commitment actually carries a lot of psychological weight with it. That is why people follow through with commitments made to others or in public and why it is important for you to commit to study with a buddy.

Plus the company never hurts either. Chances are you will both motivate each other to do more than you would have done alone.

The more you feel that you are not "in this alone" the more relaxed and confident you will be and the more you will get done.

Note: IMPORTANT**** *Study with a positive minded person. Don't get stuck listening to negative people and their excuses why they can't do this or that. These people are always looking to drag other people "down to their level" and are always reluctant to change to better themselves.*

If you arrange to study with a buddy and the person starts making negative comments... get out now! Don't waist your time trying to bring them up or convert them to your way of thinking.... it won't work! Stay positive and spend your time studying... not counseling. Leave that to the professionals.

Develop Your Concentration

Concentration is described as "intense mental application; complete attention".

It is your minds ability to focus on the task at hand and block out all other influences and distractions. To concentrate on one thing and one thing exclusively... the exam.

Information Retention

Your ability to concentrate is vital to your exam success. The more you concentrate on the subject materials the better you will retain and recall the information when the time comes to perform.

When you concentrate solely on the material it allows you less time to worry about other "stressors" or to give time for negative thoughts to enter in. And negative thoughts will try to work their way in. Self doubt is something that can be destructive so don't give your mind an opportunity to entertain negative thoughts.

For you to perform your best, all attention must be on the study material and the exam. This deep level of concentration will help you maximize your study time. In most cases, the better you can concentrate during your study time the less study time you will actually have to schedule. The saying "quality over quantity" applies to exam preparation too!

I mean... really, who wants to study for 5 hours at one sitting when you can study for 2 hours, with a high level of concentration and focus, and get the same results. No one. **Study Smarter, Not Longer!**

Benefits

Training your mind to concentrate on the task at hand will keep positive thoughts flowing and block out negative thoughts. Think of your mind as a bowl. You can only put so much in a bowl. So the more positive thoughts you put into the bowl the less room there is for negative ones.

Some of the benefits of increasing your level of concentration included:

- Peace of mind

- Self confidence

- Inner strength

- Ability to focus your mind

- Increased memory

- Ability to study and comprehend more quickly

- Less study time

Exercises

Here are some exercises to help you develop your concentration.

1) Select one thought and concentrate on it for ten minutes. This will be difficult at first but the more you do it the easier it will be to block out all other thoughts and concentrate on the one thought you have chosen.

2) Count the words in a paragraph. Count them again to ensure accuracy. Once you have completed this, count several paragraphs and then an entire page.

3) Take an object such as a spoon, fork, or anything out of a drawer. Try to concentrate on the object without mentally describing the object in words. Just focus on the object from all directions.

4) Draw a circle and color it in with any color. Now focus on the object and try not to think of any words, just focus on the object for several minutes.

5) Lie down and relax all your muscles. Once you are completely relaxed concentrated on your heartbeat and imagine your blood flowing throughout your body. After several minutes you should be able to feel the blood moving through your veins.

6) Watch the second hand on a clock. Focus just on the second hand and nothing else. Do this for two to three minutes and fight off the urge to let any other thoughts interfere with your concentration.

7) Close your eyes and visualize the number one. Say the number "one" in your head once you visualize it clearly. Now let it go and focus on the number two and repeat the process up to ten.

8) Take a coin out of your pocket. Relax every muscle in your body and concentrate on the coin and only the coin. View everything about it, its shape, color, material makeup nicks, words. Now close your eyes and visualize the coin in full detail. If you can not visualize the coin in full detail open your eyes and try again.

9) Sit in a chair and relax. Focus on a spot on the wall and release all other thoughts from your mind. Now while looking at the spot on the wall focus on your breathing. Breath in slowly and then exhale slowly. Do this for several minutes.

10) Read an article in the newspaper. Capture the essentials of the article. Now describe the article in as few words as possible to a friend or just aloud to yourself.

Learning to concentrate fully on the task at hand is difficult but the benefits are enormous. It is easy to let your mind wander off and loose your train of thought during an exam.

The better your concentration is during your exam preparation the better your exam scores will be. It is as simple as that.

Concentration is critical, specially towards the end of the exam when it is easy to get distracted and lose focus as you start to get tired.

This is when this training will pay off. You <u>will</u> remain focused and keep your concentration though the entire exam.

Note: IMPORTANT**** *These exercises are not for everyone, however, they are a valuable tool when learning to increase your concentration and mental focus.*

Try to do the exercises every other day. You will notice an increase in your information retention and recall. Plus this will help you study more efficiently and effectively!

Power of Positive Thinking

Positive thinking can reduce stress, improve your overall health, and make you much more interesting and fun to be around.

Although it is unclear exactly why positive thinkers experience health benefits, one of the theories is it helps them deal with stressful situations better. They are thinking of the best outcome, not the worst outcome, and this creates less stress and anxiety. This is better for the mind and the body.

I'll never forget an acquaintance of mine way back in the mid 80's who would shoot down new ideas like clay pigeons. Whenever a new idea would come up he would spend three times the intellectual effort to shoot it down than to consider if it would ever work. In his eyes "it would never work" no matter what it was.

Does that guy sound familiar to you? My guess is he probably does. You might have one or several people like this in your life right now. The best thing you can do is run... run... run.

I have nothing against shooting holes in a new idea to see if it stands the test of scrutiny, but just to dismiss a new idea because it represents change is unhealthy.

Negative people will try with all their might to bring you down. To make you surrender your positive "can do" attitude and keep them company in their pool of negativity. Don't let them!

Glass Half Full or Empty

Are you a "glass half full" or "glass half empty" type of person? Answering this question is a good way to find out if you are an optimist or a pessimist.

If you always see the good side of things (glass half full) then you are an optimist. If not, then you are a pessimist.

Optimists (or positive people) always consider the "what if it could work" side of things. They are happy and easy with a smile. They give as much positive energy as they get from others and are usually interesting and fun to be around.

An optimist is more likely to be successful too. They "will their self to victory". They tell THEMSELVES they can do something and this starts the ball of positivity and success rolling. Just as a snowball rolling down a mountain starts small, once it gains momentum there is little way to stop it.

Self Talk

Why is self talk important? Well, the mind is always thinking and creating "self-talk". Self-talk is the endless stream of thoughts that run through your head.

Self-talk is based on information, reason, logic, and prior experience. Self-talk also comes from misconceptions created because of misinformation or lack of information. This can be negative or positive, depending on your outlook.

For example, if someone asked you to jump over a hurdle and you've never jumped over a hurdle before, your mind would tell you either "you can do this" or "no way you can do this". This is commonly referred to as self-talk.

"PROGRAM THE VOICE INSIDE YOUR HEAD. IT WILL LISTEN, YOU OWN IT."

Programing your self talk will help you control the way you look at things and the attitude you have towards them. Self-talk is enormously powerful and you want to have it on your side.

A good example of the power of self-talk became apparent to me while working out several years ago and its power and control made a lasting impression on me.

In 1998 I started to lap swim at the local YMCA. I started to lap swim for several reasons. First, to lose weight that had accumulated over years of sitting behind a desk and remaining inactive. And second, to relieve some of the stress that comes with an upper level management job that I had been promoted to several years before.

The process of building up to a meaningful workout was slow at first, only a swimming a few laps per session. But over time I had built up to swimming 27 laps (which equalled 3/4 of a mile) per session.

I stayed at that level for many years, mainly because I could get my workout in over an hour long lunch break. But a funny thing happened several years ago when I finally went to work for myself. And it was all brought to light while talking to fellow lap swimmer at the local YMCA.

Through conversation she asked "how far do you swim each day". I said "3/4 of a mile". She asked, "why don't you just swim a mile"? "I don't know" I replied. "I have been doing this for years and never gave it much thought".

The next time in the pool I tried to swim a mile (36 laps) and around lap number twenty my mind began telling me I was tired and it was almost time to quit.

And sure enough, at lap twenty seven I was in no position to go any further. I was done. My mind had convinced my body that 3/4 of a mile was enough for today.

It was hard to believe that my body just started to feel exhausted around the 3/4 mile mark, knowing full well I could swim more laps. So the next day I decided to control my self-talk and tell myself "I am going to swim thirty six laps today" and "I could do anything I put my mind to". I was literally trying to trick myself into thinking I could swim a full mile.

Swimming a full mile was not a problem that day because my mind was reinforcing the belief that I could swim a mile. By controlling my self-talk and keeping the self-talk positive instead of negative I was able to control the outcome and achieve more than what my mind had previously programed me to accept as my unconscious limit.

I have also used this technique to swim two miles in one session and lose over 60 lbs. Controlling your self-talk is powerful, and it works.

Unconscious Limits

Your mind sets unconscious limits for everything that you do based on previous experience and other inputs of information such as things you read or discuss with others. Your mind processes all this information to set predetermined limits for you.

This was exceptionally powerful when world class runners were trying to break the four minute mile mark. It was generally thought that no one could ever run a mile under four minutes.

And for years no one could surpass that mark until May 6th, 1954. Sir Roger Bannister ran a mile in 3:59. Until that day no one had ever recorded running a mile under four minutes.

How strong was that unconscious limit? So strong that it only took _**46 days**_ for the record to be broken. The unconscious limit had been stripped away, and in only 46 days another runner achieved what only one man had ever achieved before. The sub four minute mile.

The same applies to your exam preparation. Remove your unconscious limits and give your mind the freedom to perform the way it is capable of. Learning to channel self-talk in a positive direction can help you achieve more than you ever imagined.

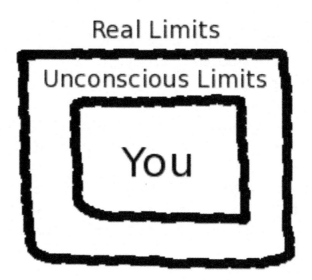

Train Your Mind

In the end, the mind will do what you train it to do. For example, do you ever catch yourself saying subconsciously that you *can't* do something? Of course you have. We all have. That is because we haven't trained our minds to accept the challenge of the task we want to perform.

It is our job to change the way we think. Think positive thoughts. "I CAN do this". "I am the best". "I will pass the exam". Train your mind to think positively and this will reduce your stress level and give you a confident feeling going into the exam.

Do not let others, or your surroundings, dictate your mental state of mind. YOU have the ultimate control and YOU control whether you think positive or negative thoughts.

This takes time and it is something that should be practiced daily. Do not think you can think positive once and everything will occur as you would like it. It just doesn't work that way. Even when you fail, resist the urge to be negative. Everything worthwhile takes some effort. But over time this will work in your favor.

You have to remember you are potentially trying to undo years of "I CAN"T" programming. Years of people telling you "YOU CAN'T" and "NO" and "IT WILL NEVER WORK".

Those are powerful messages built in to your mind. We have all heard them for many years and now is the time to turn it around.

The first "YES I CAN", and "I CAN DO WHATEVER I PUT MY MIND TO" will begin the change. It will start the little snowball rolling down the mountain... and with a little momentum comes massive change!

Self Confidence

Confidence shows in everything you do. From how you look at life to how you treat others. Confident people are people who take action. Confident people are the "doers" in the world. The people who look for ways for things to work rather than look for ways for things to fail.

Confidence is not arrogance. Confidence comes from taking decisive action and not from the outcome of that action. Confident people do not shy away from taking action because they are afraid of a failed outcome. They take action and are undaunted by the prospect of failure.

Arrogance, however, is exactly the opposite. Arrogance does not come from taking action, it comes from the result of the action. Arrogance highlights achievements and hides failures never learning anything from either.

An arrogant person is defined, in their own mind, by both their accomplishments and failures and will shy away from taking action because of the prospect of failure.

Developing Confidence

Confidence is developed through a series of "wins" or "achievements". It is developed through facing your fears and overcoming them. This gives you strength and confidence in your ability to overcome. The more you overcome, the more confident you become.

So how do you build confidence in your ability to pass an exam? Simple.... preparation! Face your fears head on and take action. Prepare every day until you know you are going to pass... there is not doubt!

Review the study material over and over again and build your level of confidence. There is no substitute for hard work and hard work builds confidence.

Have you ever seen a person walk into a room and everyone pays attention? They have a certain confidence about them that radiates form within.

They are not the wealthiest in the room. Nor the most attractive person. But this inner confidence puts them at ease when everyone else may be timid or afraid to step out of their comfort zone.

Confidence and the Exam

Your confidence will have a direct effect on your exam results. If you are confident in your ability to pass the exam it lowers your stress level and opens your mind for clearer thinking. When you project confidence your body reacts differently to circumstances. It gives you the calmness to perform at a high level.

Confidence only comes through preparation. The more you prepare, the more confident you will be in your ability to ace your exam.
This is the type of confidence you must have when you walk into the exam. An undeniable belief that you will pass the exam because of your preparation, determination, and hard work.

Nothing will stand in your way from achieving your goal!

"YOU GAIN STRENGTH, COURAGE AND CONFIDENCE BY EVERY EXPERIENCE IN WHICH YOU STOP TO LOOK FEAR IN THE FACE. YOU ARE ABLE TO SAY TO YOURSELF, 'I HAVE LIVED THROUGH THIS HORROR. I CAN TAKE THE NEXT THING THAT COMES ALONG.' YOU MUST DO THE THING YOU THINK YOU CANNOT DO."

ELEANOR ROOSEVELT

Sleep and Nutrition

The final piece of the puzzle to reducing stress is proper sleep and nutrition. Your body and mind can only function at its highest level if you give it proper rest and proper nutrition (fuel).

Your body and mind needs time to rest and good food to perform. This is easy to overlook and many times it is the first thing you sacrifice when you are preparing for an exam.

You can do everything else right to reduce stress and prepare for an exam but failing to get proper rest and nutrition could cause it all to go to waste.

Once you think about it you can see why these are essential ingredients (no pun intended) to successful exam preparation.

Sleep

Why is sleep so important? Because it is the only time your body has a chance to recharge.

A good sleep regiment should consist of at least six hours of sleep each night so your body and mind are fresh and ready to go the next morning. Anything less an you will not be fully rested and your performance will suffer because of it.

Stress can also impact sleep patterns to a point that is unhealthy. Stress related sleep disorders are fairly common and can have a major impact on your exam performance.

How many times have you tried to solve work or family related problems well into the night. Sometimes it just cannot be avoided but trying to leave work at work and going to bed with a clear mind will leave you refreshed and ready to tackle the problems of the day when the next day arrives.

To get a better nights sleep try these simple tips to reduce stress and rest up.

1) List problems bothering you with possible solutions before bed.

2) Put work into perspective. When work is over, leave it. Turn it off.

3) Designate cell free time. Even if it is only a half hour or during dinner.

4) Never check work email before bed.

5) Try to simplify one thing each day.

6) Grab a nap if you can. Sleep reduces stress hormones.

7) Laugh! Laughter reduces stress and raises <u>anti-stress</u> hormones making it easier to fall asleep.

8) Owning a pets can significantly lower your heart rate and blood pressure letting you rest longer.

9) Hug a family member. Affection reduces stress and makes it easier to sleep.

10) Take a fifteen minute walk. Exercise is the <u>BEST</u> stress reliever and you will be ready to sleep when the time comes!

These tips can make it easier to get a good nights rest and ready to go in the morning.

Nutrition

Proper nutrition to reduce stress you say? Yes, it's true! Proper nutrition plays a key role in our body's performance and ability to rest.

There is plenty of information about the ties between nutrition and sleep. One of my favorite articles is called "Sleep Deeper with Better Nutrition". It covers a mound of information about protein "super foods" and herbs that will help you get a better nights rest naturally.

Some of the "super foods" are items such as green tea, buffalo, walnuts, sardines, artichokes, kiwis, dark chocolate, cherries, and many others. These foods supply the body with super fuel and burn very efficiently so you don't feel full or tired after eating them.

I prefer making adjustments to diet over prescription drugs or other methods because it is natural and enhances the body's ability to rest.

Food or drink that contain sugar or caffeine can give you a temporary boost but the crash won't help you towards the end of the exam when you typically need it the most so try to avoid these.

What If I Fail

The most successful people fail all the time! It is a result of taking action. There is no shame in failure, only shame in not getting back up, learning from your mistakes, and trying again.

Golf legend Jack Nicklaus used to welcome a bad golf hole or two each round because the sooner he got them out of the way the sooner he could move on and make the round a great one. He embraced temporary failure as part of being successful.

Truthfully, the more you fail the closer you are to succeeding as long as you learn from your mistakes. Few people succeed without failing many times first. It's a learning process and failure is one of the steps. You can say failure is the downpayment on success and it really is. Chances are good you will fail before you succeed but don't let it define you or hold you back. Expect it and learn from it. If you don't fail it shows you haven't taken action and just sat on the sidelines and that is the worst fate of all.

Overcome your fear of failure and success will be yours. Nothing will stand in your way. Preparation is the key. If you have prepared properly you will not fail. But if you should, embrace it, be accountable for it, and start again with more resolve than ever.

The highway is littered with people who have failed. Everyone fails. The people who win get right back on the horse and start riding again.

"I HAVE NOT FAILED. I'VE JUST FOUND 10,000 WAYS THAT WON'T WORK."

THOMAS EDISON

Getting Help

Is there a certain section of material that is just not making sense or sinking in? GET HELP! Don't wait or, worse yet, be too shy to ask for help. Search out help as fast as you can. Now is not the time to be shy or hesitate to ask for assistance.

Many teachers and instructors are more than willing to give you a helping hand. That is their profession and most of them generally love to help people. Take advantage of their help if you need it.

REMEMBER, YOU ARE NOT IN THIS ALONE!

Reaching out for help and getting it will give you a feeling of accomplishment and confidence. That confidence will be your friend and something you want to continually build upon as you ready yourself for your exam.

"ONE IMPORTANT KEY TO SUCCESS IS SELF-CONFIDENCE. AN IMPORTANT KEY TO SELF- CONFIDENCE IS PREPARATION."

ARTHUR ASHE

Common Anatomical Terminology

Anatomy terminology can seem complex and overwhelming when just starting out. Once you familiarize yourself with some of the more common terms it will make your preparation much easier. Just like anything else, it will take practice. Learn and few terms each day and before you know it you will have established a good base to work from.

Take time to familiarize yourself with these terms to make you a better medical coder.

Anatomy Terminology - Number	
Term	**Meaning**
mono-, uni-	one
bi	two
tri	three

Anatomy Terminology - Direction and Position

Term	Meaning
ab-	away from
ad-	toward
ecto-, exo-	outside
endo-	inside
epi-	upon
anterior or ventral	at or near the front surface of the body
posterior or dorsal	at or near the real surface of the body
superior	above
inferior	below
lateral	side
distal	farthest from center
proximal	nearest to center

Anatomy Terminology - Basic Terms

Term	Meaning
abdominal	abdomen
buccal	cheek
cranial	skull
digital	fingers and toes
femoral	thigh
gluteal	buttocks
hallux	great toe
inguinal	groin
lumbar	lowest part of spine
mammary	breast
nasal	nose
occipital	back of head
pectoral	breastbone
thoracic	chest
umbilical	navel
ventral	belly

Anatomy Terminology - Conditions - Prefixes

Term	Meaning
ambi-	both
dys-	bad, painful, difficult
eu-	good, normal
homo-	same
iso-	equal, same
mal-	bad, poor

Anatomy Terminology - Conditions - Suffixes

Term	Meaning
-algia	pain
-emia	blood
-itis	inflamation
-lysis	destruction, breakdown
-oid	like
-opathy	disease of
-pnea	breathing

Anatomy Terminology - Surgical Procedures

Term	Meaning
-centesis	puncture a cavity to remove fluid
-ectomy	surgical removal or excision
-ostomy	a new permanent opening
-otomy	cutting into, incision
-opexy	surgical fixation
-oplasty	surgical repair
-otripsy	crushing or destroying

Medical Terminology Prefix, Root, and Suffixes

Being familiar with Medical Terminology prefixes, roots and suffixes are essential for a medical coder. This illustrates how roots, prefixes, and suffixes are used to denote number or size, direction, color, anatomical locations, as well as other meanings.

Take time to familiarize yourself with these terms to make you a better medical coder.

Medical Terminology - Prefixes and Roots Denoting Number or Size	
Term	**Meaning**
bi-	two
dipl/o	two, double
hemi-	half
hyper-	over or more than usual
hypo-	under or less than usual
iso-	equal, same
macro-	large
megal/o-	enlargement
micro-	small
mono-	one
multi-	many
nulli-	none
poly-	many
semi-	half, partial

Medical Terminology - Prefixes and Roots Denoting Number or Size	
tri-	three
uni-	one

Medical Terminology - Roots Denoting Color	
Term	**Meaning**
chlor/o	green
cyan/o	blue
erythr/o	red
leuk/o	white
melan/o	black
xanth/o	yellow

Medical Terminology - Prefixes and Roots Denoting Relative Direction

Term	Meaning
per-	through
peri-	around
post-	behind, after
poster/o	behind
pre-	before, in front of
pro-	before
retr/o	behind, in back of
sub-	under
super-	beyond
supra-	above
syn-	together
trans-	across
ventr/o	belly

Medical Terminology - Roots Denoting Anatomical Location

Term	Meaning
abdomin/o	abdomen
acr/o	extremity
aden/o	gland
angi/o	vessel
arter/i/o	artery
arthr/o	joint
blast/o	embryo
blephar/o	eyelid
bronch/i/o	bronchus
calcane/o	calaneous
cardi/o	heart
carp/o	carpal, wrist
cephal/o	head
cerebr/o	cerebrum
cheil/o	lip
chol/e	bile, gall
chondr/o	cartilage
cocc/i	coccus
col/o	colon
colp/o	vagina

Medical Terminology - Roots Denoting Anatomical Location

Term	Meaning
condyl/o	condyle
core/o, cor/o	pupil
corne/o	cornea
cost/o	ribs
crani/o	cranium
cycl/o	ciliary body
cyst/o	bladder, sac
cyt/o	cell
dactyl/o	fingers or toes
dent/o	tooth
derm/o	skin
dermat/o	skin
duoden/o	duodenum
enter/o	intestine
esophag/o	esophagus
fibr/o	fiber
gangli/o	ganglion
gastr/o	stomach
gingiv/o	gums
gloss/o	tongue

Medical Terminology - Roots Denoting Anatomical Location

Term	Meaning
gynec/o	women
hem/o, hemat/o	blood
hepat/o	liver
hidr/o	sweat
humer/o	humerus
hydr/o	water
hyster/o	uterus
ile/o	ileum
irid/o, ir/o	iris
ischi/o	ischium
jejun/o	jejunum
kerat/o	cornea
lacrim/o	tear
laryng/o	larynx
lip/o	fat
lith/o	stone, calculus
lumb/o	loin, lumbar area
ment/o	chin
my/o	muscle
myel/o	spinal cord, bone marrow

Medical Terminology - Roots Denoting Anatomical Location

Term	Meaning
nas/o	nose
nephr/o	kidney
neur/o	nerve
omphal/o	umbilicus, navel
onych/o	nail
oophor/o	ovary
opthalm/o	eye
orchid/o	testicles
oste/o	bone
ot/o	ear
pancreat/o	pancreas
pely/i	pelvis
peps/o/ia	digestion
phalang/o	phalange
pharyng/o	pharynx
phas/o	speech
phleb/o	veins
pleur/o	pleura
pne/o	air, breathing
pneum/o, pneumono	lung

Medical Terminology - Roots Denoting Anatomical Location

Term	Meaning
pod/o	foot
proct/o	rectum, anus
psych/o	mind
pub/o	pubis
py/o	pus
pyel/o	kidney
rect/o	rectum
ren/o	kidney
retin/o	retina
rhin/o	nose
salping/o	fallopian tube
scler/o	sclera
spermat/o	sperm
splen/o	spleen
stern/o	sternum, breastbone
stomat/o	mouth
thorac/o	thorax, chest
trache/o	trachea
traumat/o	tramua
tympan/o	eardrum

Medical Terminology - Roots Denoting Anatomical Location

Term	Meaning
ur/o	urine
ureter/o	ureter
urethr/o	urethra
vas/o	vessel
viscer/o	gut, contents of the abdomen

Medical Terminology - Other Prefixes

Term	Meaning
a-, an-	without
anti-	against
auto-	self
brady-	slow
con-	with
contra-	against
dis-	free of
dys-	difficult or without pain
mal-	bad, poor
neo-	new
syn-	together
tachy-	fast

Medical Terminology - Other Roots

Term	Meaning
necr/o	dead
noct/i	night
par/o	bear
phag/o	eat
phil/o	attraction
plast/o	repair, formation
pyr/o	fire, fever
scler/o	tough, hard
sinistr/o	left
syphil/o	syphilis
therap/o	treatment
therm/o	heat
thromb/o	thrombosis
troph/o	development

Medical Terminology - Other Suffixes

Term	Meaning
algia	pain
ar	pertaining to
centesis	puncture
clysis	irrigation
ectasia	dilatation, dilation
ectomy	excision
emes/is	vomiting
emia	blood
esthesia	feelings
genesis, gen/o	development, formation, beginning
gnosis	know
ia	noun ending
ia, ic	pertaining to
it is	inflammation
manual	hand
meter	measuring intrument
oid	resembling
ologist	one who studies
ology	study of
oma	tumor

Medical Terminology - Other Suffixes

Term	Meaning
opia	vision
orrhagia	hemorrhage
orrhaphy	suture
orrhea	flow
orrhexis	rupture
osis	condition of
ostomy	new opening
otomy	incision
pedal	foot
pexy	fixing, fixation
phob/ia	fear
plasm	growth
plegia, plegic	paralysis
ptosis	drooping
scope, scopy	examining, looking at
spasm	twitching
sperm	sperm
stasis	slow, stop
tome	intrument
tripsy	crushing

Notes

Notes

Notes

Notes

Resources

One of the most difficult challenges of taking the medical coding certification exam is finishing it in the allotted time. We have heard this from hundreds of students and medical coders. We've created a course to address this problem specifically. It is the Medical Coding Exam System. If you are finding it difficult to finish the exam on time, don't take a chance on failing. Invest in sharpening your exam time management skills and pass the exam the first time.

Exam Preparation Products We Recommend

Medical Coding Exam Prep Course
http://medicalcodingpro.com/medical-coding-certification-prep-course/

Medical Coding Exam System
http://medicalcodingexamsystem.com

Faster Coder - Code Faster - Code Better
http://fastercoder.com

Other Resources

Elite Members Area – 7 day FREE trial!
http://medicalcodingpromembers.com

Medical Coding Pro – main website
http://medicalcodingpro.com

MEDICAL CODING PRO

Medical Coding Pro provides information about medical coding. We also help people in the medical coding community prepare for the medical coding certification exam.

Our mission is to help everyone we can pass the exam and gain their certification as quickly as possible. To do this we offer quality exam preparation tools such as Medical Coding Practice Exams, the Medical Coding Exam System, the Medical Coding Exam Strategy and the Medical Coding Pro Elite Members Area.

Visit us on the web at:

www.MedicalCodingPro.com

www.MedicalCodingProMembers.com

www.MedicalCodingExamSystem.com

www.MedicalCodingNews.org

CPSIA information can be obtained
at www.ICGtesting.com
Printed in the USA
LVOW02s0413040817
543805LV00006B/348/P